Obstetric and Gynecologic Emergencies

Editors

SUSAN E. DANTONI
PETER J. PAPADAKOS

CRITICAL CARE CLINICS

www.criticalcare.theclinics.com

Consulting Editor
RICHARD W. CARLSON

January 2016 • Volume 32 • Number 1

ELSEVIER

1600 John F. Kennedy Boulevard ● Suite 1800 ● Philadelphia, Pennsylvania, 19103-2899

http://www.theclinics.com

CRITICAL CARE CLINICS Volume 32, Number 1
January 2016 ISSN 0749-0704, ISBN-13: 978-0-323-41445-6

Editor: Patrick Manley
Developmental Editor: Casey Jackson

Critical Care Clinics (ISSN: 0749-0704) is published quarterly by Elsevier Inc., 360 Park Avenue South, New York, NY 10010-1710. Months of issue are January, April, July, and October. Business and Editorial Offices: 1600 John F. Kennedy Blvd., Suite 1800, Philadelphia, PA 19103-2899. Customer Service Office: 6277 Sea Harbor Drive, Orlando, FL 32887-4800. Periodicals postage paid at New York, NY and additional mailing offices. Subscription prices are $215.00 per year for US individuals, $551.00 per year for US institution, $100.00 per year for US students and residents, $255.00 per year for Canadian individuals, $691.00 per year for Canadian institutions, $300.00 per year for international individuals, $691.00 per year for international institutions and $150.00 per year for Canadian and foreign students/residents. To receive student/resident rate, orders must be accompanied by name of affiliated institution, date of term, and the signature of program/residency coordinator on institution letterhead. Orders will be billed at individual rate until proof of status is received. Foreign air speed delivery is included in all *Clinics* subscription prices. All prices are subject to change without notice. POSTMASTER: Send address changes to *Critical Care Clinics*, Elsevier Periodicals Customer Service, 11830 Westline Industrial Drive, St. Louis, MO 63146. **Customer Service: 1-800-654-2452 (US). From outside of the US, call 1-314-447-8871. Fax: 1-314-447-8029. E-mail: journalscustomerservice-usa@ elsevier.com (for print support) or journalsonlinesupport-usa@elsevier.com (for online support).**

Reprints. For copies of 100 or more of articles in this publication, please contact the Commercial Reprints Department, Elsevier Inc., 360 Park Avenue South, New York, NY 10010-1710. Tel.: 212-633-3874; Fax: 212-633-3820; E-mail: reprints@elsevier.com.

Critical Care Clinics is also published in Spanish by Editorial Inter-Medica, Junin 917, 1er A, 1113, Buenos Aires, Argentina.

Critical Care Clinics is covered in *MEDLINE/PubMed (Index Medicus), EMBASE/Excerpta Medica, Current Concepts/ Clinical Medicine, ISI/BIOMED,* and *Chemical Abstracts.*

Contributors

CONSULTING EDITOR

RICHARD W. CARLSON, MD, PhD
Chairman Emeritus, Director, Medical Intensive Care Unit, Department of Medicine, Maricopa Medical Center; Professor, University of Arizona College of Medicine; Professor, Department of Medicine, Mayo Graduate School of Medicine, Phoenix, Arizona; Mayo Clinic, Scottsdale, Arizona

EDITORS

SUSAN E. DANTONI, MD, FACOG
OB Hospitalist, Surgical Director OB Family Practice Fellowship, Bellevue Women's Center/Ellis Hospital, Schenectady, New York; Clinical Assistant Professor, Albany Medical College, Albany, New York

PETER J. PAPADAKOS, MD, FCCM, FAARC
Director of Critical Care Medicine; Professor Anesthesiology, Surgery, Neurology and Neurosurgery; Department of Anesthesiology, University of Rochester School of Medicine, University of Rochester Medical Center, Rochester, New York

AUTHORS

NYIMA ALI, MD
Attending Staff Physician, Department of Obstetrics and Gynecology, Maricopa Integrated Health System, District Medical Group, Phoenix, Arizona

STEPHEN J. BACAK, DO, MPH
Fellow and Clinical Instructor, Division of Maternal-Fetal Medicine, University of Rochester Medical Center, Rochester, New York

ARI BALOFSKY, MD
Department of Anesthesiology, University of Rochester Medical Center, Rochester, New York

RICHARD W. CARLSON, MD, PhD
Chairman Emeritus, Director, Medical Intensive Care Unit, Department of Medicine, Maricopa Medical Center; Professor, University of Arizona College of Medicine; Professor, Department of Medicine, Mayo Graduate School of Medicine, Phoenix, Arizona; Mayo Clinic, Scottsdale, Arizona

AHMAD CHEBBO, MD
Maricopa Medical Center, Phoenix, Arizona

DEAN V. COONROD, MD, MPH
Attending Staff Physician and Chair, Department of Obstetrics and Gynecology, Maricopa Integrated Health System, District Medical Group; Executive Chair and Professor, Department of Obstetrics and Gynecology, University of Arizona College of Medicine, Phoenix, Arizona

MAURICIO RUIZ CUERO, MD
Fellow, Neurocritical Care, Henry Ford Hospital, Detroit, Michigan

SUSAN E. DANTONI, MD, FACOG
OB Hospitalist, Surgical Director OB Family Practice Fellowship, Bellevue Women's Center/Ellis Hospital, Schenectady, New York; Clinical Assistant Professor, Albany Medical College, Albany, New York

MAKSIM FEDARAU, MD
Assistant Professor, Department of Anesthesiology, University of Rochester Medical Center, Rochester, New York

AMIE HOEFNAGEL, MD
Assistant Professor of Anesthesiology, University of Rochester, Rochester, New York

HUAYONG HU, MD
Department of Anesthesiology, Yale New Haven Hospital, New Haven, Connecticut

ANNA KAMINSKI, DO
Assistant Professor of Anesthesiology, University of Rochester, Rochester, New York

MARCIN KARCZ, MD, MSc
Department of Anesthesiology, University of Rochester School of Medicine, Rochester, New York

CHRISTELLE KASSIS, MD
Maricopa Medical Center, Phoenix, Arizona

AMIE LUCIA, DO
Clinical Assistant Professor, SUNY Upstate Medical University, Syracuse, New York

THOMAS R. McCORMICK, DMin
Department Bioethics and Humanities, Senior Lecturer Emeritus, University of Washington, Seattle, Washington

MARIO MENK, MD
Department of Anesthesiology and Intensive Care Medicine, Charité - University Medicine Berlin, Berlin, Germany

COURTNEY OLSON-CHEN, MD
Division of Maternal-Fetal Medicine, Department of Obstetrics and Gynecology, University of Rochester Medical Center, Rochester, New York

PETER J. PAPADAKOS, MD, FCCM, FAARC
Director of Critical Care Medicine; Professor Anesthesiology, Surgery, Neurology and Neurosurgery; Department of Anesthesiology, University of Rochester School of Medicine, University of Rochester Medical Center, Rochester, New York

IOANA PASCA, MD
Department of Anesthesiology, Loma Linda University Medical Center, Loma Linda, California

DAVID SCHWAIBERGER, MD
Department of Anesthesiology and Intensive Care Medicine, Charité - University Medicine Berlin, Berlin, Germany

NEIL S. SELIGMAN, MD, MS
Division of Maternal-Fetal Medicine, Department of Obstetrics and Gynecology, University of Rochester Medical Center, Rochester, New York

LESLIE TAMURA, DO
Maricopa Medical Center, Phoenix, Arizona; Advocate Lutheran General Hospital, Park Ridge, Illinois

SUSANNA TAN, MD
Maricopa Medical Center, Phoenix, Arizona

LORALEI L. THORNBURG, MD
Associate Professor, Fellowship Program Director, Division of Maternal-Fetal Medicine, University of Rochester Medical Center, Rochester, New York

PANAYIOTIS N. VARELAS, MD, PhD
Division Head, Neurosciences Critical Care Services; Director, Neuro-Intensive Care Unit; Professor, Department of Neurology, Henry Ford Hospital, Wayne State University, Detroit, Michigan

ALBERT YU, DO
Assistant Professor of Anesthesiology, University of Rochester, Rochester, New York

Contents

Acute liver failure is a rare but life-threatening medical emergency in pregnancy whose true incidence remains unknown. Many cases of acute liver
failure are caused by pregnancy-related conditions such as acute fatty
liver of pregnancy and HELLP syndrome. However, acute deterioration
in liver function can also be caused by drug overdose, viral infections,
and an exacerbation of underlying chronic liver disease. This article provides an overview of the normal liver changes that occur during pregnancy,
and summarizes the most common conditions and general management
strategies of liver failure during pregnancy.

Renal failure during pregnancy affects both mother and fetus, and may be
related to preexisting disease or develop secondary to diseases of pregnancy. Causes include hypovolemia, sepsis, shock, preeclampsia, thrombotic microangiopathies, and renal obstruction. Treatment focuses on
supportive measures, while pharmacologic treatment is viewed as
second-line therapy, and is more useful in mitigating harmful effects than
treating the underlying cause. When supportive measures and pharmacotherapy prove inadequate, dialysis may be required, with the goal being
to prolong pregnancy until delivery is feasible. Outcomes and recommendations depend primarily on the underlying cause.

Fewer than 2% of all peripartal patients need intensive care unit admission.
However, due to some anatomic and physiologic changes in pregnancy,
respiratory failure can be promoted. This article reviews several obstetric
and nonobstetric diseases that lead to respiratory failure and the treatment
of these. Furthermore, invasive and noninvasive ventilation in pregnancy is
discussed and suggestions of medication during ventilation are given.

Management of peripartum heart disease in the intensive care unit requires
optimization of maternal hemodynamics and maintenance of fetal perfusion. This requires fetal monitoring and should address the parturient's oxygen saturation, hemoglobin, and cardiac output as it relates to uterine
blood flow. Pharmacologic strategies have limited evidence pertaining to
hemodynamic stabilization and fetal perfusion. There is some evidence
that surgical management of critical mitral stenosis should be percutaneous
when possible because cardiac bypass is associated with increased fetal
mortality. Fetal monitoring strategies should address central organ perfusion because peripheral scalp pH has not been associated with improved
fetal outcomes.

Trauma continues to be a leading cause of nonobstetric maternal and fetal mortality worldwide. Caring for the pregnant trauma patient requires a systematic and multidisciplinary approach. It is important to understand the anatomic and physiologic changes that occur during pregnancy. Accepted trauma guidelines for imaging and interventions should generally not be deviated from just because a patient is pregnant. Focus should be placed on injury prevention and education of at risk patients to decrease the morbidity and mortality associated with traumatic injuries in pregnant patients.

The year 2015 marked the 200th anniversary of the birth of Ignaz Semmelweis, the Hungarian physician who identified unhygienic practices of physicians as a major cause of childbed fever or puerperal sepsis. Although such practices have largely disappeared as a factor in the development of chorioamnionitis and postpartum or puerperal endometritis, it is appropriate that this article on sepsis in pregnancy acknowledges his contributions to maternal health. This review describes the incidence and mortality of sepsis in pregnancy, methods to identify and define sepsis in this population, including scoring systems, causes, and sites of infection during pregnancy and parturition and management guidelines.

Ethical issues that arise in the care of pregnant women are challenging to physicians, especially in critical care situations. By familiarizing themselves with the concepts of medical ethics in obstetrics, physicians will become more capable of approaching complex ethical situations with a clear and structured framework. This review discusses ethical approaches regarding 3 specific scenarios: (1) the life of the fetus versus the life of the mother and situations of questionable maternal decision making; (2) withdrawal of care in a brain-dead pregnant patient; and (3) domestic violence and the pregnant patient.

CRITICAL CARE CLINICS

THE CLINICS ARE AVAILABLE ONLINE!
Access your subscription at:
www.theclinics.com

Preface

Obstetrics and Gynecology Emergencies

 CrossMark

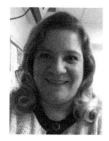   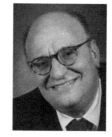

Susan E. Dantoni, MD, FACOG   Peter J. Papadakos, MD, FCCM, FAARC
Editors

This issue of *Critical Care Clinics* featuring Obstetrics and Gynecologic Emergencies began 20 years ago when a rather new obstetrician found herself knee deep in trouble with a patient experiencing an amniotic fluid embolism. Fortunately, the critical care team led by a very experienced intensivist arrived quickly, and because a multidisciplinary approach was taken, the patient experienced a very good outcome. This marriage of critical care and obstetrics led to many more collaborative efforts caring for very complicated patients. It also led to two children, three cats, a dog, a fish, and a horse, but that is another story!

While the vast majority of obstetric patients are delivered without incident, pregnancy remains a potentially high-risk condition with its own unique disease processes sometimes requiring the expertise of a multitude of clinicians. It is just as vital for the obstetrician to be educated regarding these medical complications as it is for other specialists, especially intensivists, to be aware of the pathophysiologic processes of pregnancy that may complicate the medical management of very sick gravida.

We have attempted to provide a broad review of critical care problems seen in obstetrics from anesthetic management to ethical issues. We have engaged experts to discuss neurologic, cardiac, renal, and hepatic complications of pregnancy. The topic of sepsis specifically addresses the complex and sometimes difficult conditions unique to pregnancy, which account for a significant amount of maternal morbidity and mortality throughout the world. The complex trauma issues join the trauma surgeon and the obstetrician in a battle to save both the mother and the fetus. This interplay of support of both parties is at the core of this aspect of critical care.

We are hopeful that this issue of *Critical Care Clinics* in which obstetric issues are covered is of interest not only to the critical care physician but also to the obstetric physician.

Crit Care Clin 32 (2016) xi–xii
http://dx.doi.org/10.1016/j.ccc.2015.10.001
0749-0704/16/$ – see front matter © 2016 Published by Elsevier Inc.

criticalcare.theclinics.com

This work is dedicated to our two children, Yanni and Ava, who have dealt with beepers, phone calls, and missed events. We love you both and appreciate your patience and understanding of our crazy careers.

Susan E. Dantoni, MD, FACOG
Bellevue Women's Center/Ellis Hospital
Schenectady, NY, USA

Albany Medical College
Albany, NY, USA

Peter J. Papadakos, MD, FCCM, FAARC
University of Rochester
Rochester, NY, USA

E-mail addresses:
obdocsue@aol.com (S.E. Dantoni)
peter_papadakos@urmc.rochester.edu (P.J. Papadakos)

Anesthetic Complications in Pregnancy

Amie Hoefnagel, MD*, Albert Yu, DO, Anna Kaminski, DO

KEYWORDS

- Thrombocytopenia • Epidural hematoma • Aspiration • Neuraxial blockade
- Failed intubation • Postdural puncture headache • Neuropathy
- Transient neurologic symptoms

KEY POINTS

- An epidural hematoma is symptomatic bleeding within the spine whereby accumulating blood outside the dura can cause rare but potentially catastrophic compression of neural tissue by direct injury or ischemia. There is no recommended absolute minimum platelet count that would contraindicate neuraxial procedures.
- Neuraxial blockade consists of either epidural or spinal blockade, the goal of which is to provide analgesia for delivery of the infant. Common complications of neuraxial blockade include hypotension, high spinal, local anesthetic systemic toxicity, persistent neuropathy, transient neurologic symptoms, and postdural puncture headache.
- Anticoagulant use is not an absolute contraindication to neuraxial placement; however, one must know the medication dosage, frequency, and last administration. National guidelines exist to aid in providing safe care in the setting of ever-changing anticoagulation medications.
- During pregnancy, many anatomic and physiologic changes occur that can lead to difficult airway management and increased the risk of aspiration.
- In the event of maternal cardiac arrest, the patient should be positioned with left uterine tilt and prepared for delivery of the fetus via cesarean section if there is not a return of maternal circulation after 4 minutes.

THROMBOCYTOPENIA/EPIDURAL HEMATOMA

Introduction

An epidural hematoma is symptomatic bleeding within the spine where accumulating blood outside the dura can cause rare but potentially catastrophic compression of neural tissue by direct injury or ischemia. Reported rates range from 1:2600 to 1:220,000. Even though pregnancy is a prothrombotic, hypercoagulable state, a decreased number or function of platelets (ie, with pre-eclampsia or hemolysis,

Department of Anesthesiology, University of Rochester, 601 Elmwood Avenue, Rochester, NY 14642, USA
* Corresponding author.
E-mail address: amiehoefnagel@gmail.com

Crit Care Clin 32 (2016) 1–28
http://dx.doi.org/10.1016/j.ccc.2015.08.009
0749-0704/16/$ – see front matter © 2016 Elsevier Inc. All rights reserved.

elevated liver enzymes, low platelet count [HELLP] syndrome) or anticoagulant use can predispose the parturient to development of an epidural hematoma.[1,2]

Risks

In a meta-analysis of spinal epidural hematomas from 1926 to 1996, the most common cause was idiopathic; the second was anticoagulant medications; fifth was spinal/ epidural procedures with anticoagulant use, and the tenth on the list was spinal/ epidural procedure without anticoagulant.[1]

Other risk factors include

- Increased age (55–70 years old)
- History of gastrointestinal bleeding
- Aspirin use during anticoagulation
- Length of therapy
- Female gender
- Intensity of anticoagulant
- Insertion or removal of epidural catheter
- Insertion of spinal or epidural needles (**Fig. 1**)

Combination Therapies

- Vigilance, frequent neurologic monitoring after neuraxial procedures looking for excessive motor and sensory blockade
- Surgical decompression; most commonly with laminectomy and hematoma evacuation
  - Only 38% of patients had partial neurologic recovery and usually with surgery before 12 hours of symptom onset.
- Recommendations from the American Society of Anesthesiologists (ASA) practice guidelines[3–5]:
  - A specific platelet count predictive of neuraxial anesthetic complications has not been determined. The anesthesiologist's decision to order or require a platelet count should be individualized and based on a patient's history, physical examination, and clinical signs.
  - Platelet count is clinically useful for parturients with suspected pregnancy-related hypertensive disorders, such as pre-eclampsia or HELLP syndrome, and for other disorders associated with coagulopathy because it reduces maternal anesthetic complications.
  - Routine platelet count is not necessary in the healthy parturient.
  - Neuraxial anesthesia is best avoided in patients with coagulopathy, significant thrombocytopenia, platelet dysfunction, or those who have received fibrino-lytic/thrombolytic therapy (**Table 1**).

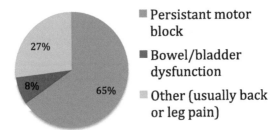

■ Persistant motor block

■ Bowel/bladder dysfunction

▨ Other (usually back or leg pain)

27%

8%

65%

Fig. 1. Initial presenting symptom. (*Data from* Kreppel D, Antoniadis G, Seeling W. Spinal hematoma: a literature survey with meta-analysis of 613 patients. Neurosurg Rev 2003;26:1–49.)

Table 1
Anticoagulation and neuraxial anesthesia/analgesia guidelines for labor and delivery[6] from the University of Michigan

Drug (Generic)	Trade Names	Dose	Time Interval for Neuraxial Procedure After Last Dose	Time Interval to Restart Medication After Catheter Is Removed
Unfractionated Heparin	Heparin	5000 units sq BID	No significant risk[a]	No significant risk
Unfractionated Heparin	Heparin	>5000 unit sq BID, any IV dose	4 h, aPTT within normal limits[a]	2 h
LMWH, Enoxaparin	Lovenox	Prophylactic dose: 40 mg sq BID 0.5 mg/kg sq BID	12 h	2 h
LMWH, Enoxaparin	Lovenox	Therapeutic dose: 1–1.5 mg/kg sq daily/BID	24 h	2 h
LMWH, Dalteparin	Fragmin	Prophylactic dose: 2500–500 units sq BID	12 h	2 h
LMWH, Dalteparin	Fragmin	Therapeutic dose: >5000 units sq BID or 100 units/kg BID	24 h	2 h
ASA	ASA, Bayer	Any dose	No significant risk	No significant risk
Warfarin	Coumadin	Any dose	3–5 d, INR <1.3	Same day

Anti-activated Factor X (anti-Xa) is used to monitor heparin levels in patients being treated with LMWH. Prophylactic dosing has peak anti-Xa activity 0.2 to 0.4 IU/mL; therapeutic dosing has peak anti-Xa activity greater than 0.5 to 1.0 IU/mL 4 h after dose.

In the case of baby ASA and another agent, follow the appropriate wait times after holding the second agent. For example, baby ASA + Lovenox 40 BID/0.5 mg/kg or less: recommended wait time after holding Lovenox is 12 h.

Abbreviations: aPTT, activated partial thromboplastin time; ASA, acetylsalicylic acid aspirin; BID, twice a day; INR, international normalized ratio; LMWH, low-molecular-weight heparin.

[a] Check platelet count if >4 days therapy.

Patient Evaluation

1. Neurologic examination
2. Neurologic imaging[7]
   a. MRI (**Table 2**)
   b. Computed tomography (CT)/CT myelography, only if MRI is unavailable

Summary Discussion

There is no recommended absolute minimum platelet count that would contraindicate neuraxial procedures; however, less than 100,000 is often quoted. More important is

Table 2
Hematoma appearance on MRI

	T1	T2
<24 h	Isodense signal	Homogenous high signal
>24 h	High signal	Same as CSF

the relative decline from baseline, rate of decline, and overall clinical picture of that patient, that is, if there are disease processes that would predispose the patient to a spinal epidural hematoma. As always, clinical decision-making and risk/benefit analysis remain key for optimum patient care.

AIRWAY
Aspiration

During pregnancy, many anatomic and physiologic changes occur that can lead to difficult airway management and increased the risk of aspiration, which can lead to chemical pneumonitis. Nearly all parturients have a gastric pH less than 2.5, and more than 60% of them have gastric volumes greater than 25 mL.[8]

Aspiration risks

- Lower esophageal sphincter (LES) displaced cephalad and anteriorly leading to incompetence
- LES tone decreased from progesterone effects
- Increased intra-abdominal pressure from gravid uterus
- Placental gastrin secretion causes hypersecretion of gastric acid
- Opioids and anticholinergics reduce LES pressure and delay gastric emptying
- Delayed gastric emptying is associated with labor pains

Patient evaluation

Regardless of the time of last oral intake, all patients are considered to have a full stomach and to be at risk for pulmonary aspiration. A thorough history to include last oral intake time and what was ingested should be done before any sedation, neuraxial procedure, or general anesthetic.[8]

ASA recommendations for aspiration prophylaxis[9]

- Oral intake of modest amounts of clear liquids may be allowed for uncomplicated laboring patients.
- The uncomplicated patient undergoing elective cesarean delivery may have modest amounts of clear liquids up to 2 hours before induction of anesthesia.
- The volume of liquid ingested is less important than the presence of particulate matter in the liquid ingested.
- Patients with additional risk factors for aspiration (eg, morbid obesity, diabetes, difficult airway) or patients at increased risk for operative delivery (eg, non-reassuring fetal heart rate pattern) may have further restrictions of oral intake, determined on a case-by-case basis.
- Solid foods should be avoided in laboring patients.
- Patients undergoing elective surgery (eg, scheduled cesarean delivery or post-partum tubal ligation) should undergo a fasting period for solids of 6 to 8 hours depending on the type of food ingested (eg, fat content).

Treatment options

Physicians should consider one or more of the medications listed in **Table 3** to mitigate aspiration pneumonitis.[10]

Summary/discussion

Because of anatomic changes associated with pregnancy, pregnant patients have an increased risk for aspiration. This aspiration may take the form of bacteria from the oropharynx (*Staphylococcus aureus*, gram-negative and or anaerobic bacteria), liquids, gastric acid, or particulate matter. Symptoms range from none to cough,

Table 3
Useful medication for mitigation of aspiration pneumonitis

Drug Class	Example with Dose and Route	Benefit
Clear nonparticulate antacid	Sodium citrate 15–30 mL orally every 3 h	Maintains gastric pH >2.5
H-2 antagonist	Ranitidine 100–150 mg orally or 50 mg IV	Reduces gastric acid volume and pH[a]
Prokinetic	Metoclopramide 10 mg orally or IV	Decreases gastric volume, increases LES tone, decreases peripartum nausea and vomiting

[a] No effect on gastric contents already present.

bronchospasm, cyanosis, tachypnea, pulmonary edema, and rarely, hypotension and hypoxemia for liquid aspiration. Treatment is primarily prevention; if that fails, the patient should be repositioned into the Trendelenburg position and oropharyngeal suction tried next. Intubation follows if the patient becomes apneic, hypoxic, or is unable to protect her airway. Once the endotracheal tube (ETT) is in place, a soft suction catheter should be passed, and the ETT should be suctioned before positive pressure ventilation is commenced to prevent pushing aspirated material further into the airspaces. If the patient has become hypoxic, there may not be time for this maneuver because oxygenation should be the primary goal. Finally, bronchoscopy, pulmonary lavage, and antibiotics are usually not necessary unless there has been aspiration of particulate matter[10] (**Fig. 2**).

Difficult Airway

Introduction
A study of the Centers for Disease Control and Prevention material mortality data showed that anesthesia-related mortality from 1979 to 2002 most often was associated with cesarean section (86%), intubation failure (23%), and respiratory failure (20%)[11] In these cases of difficult airways, the potential is not only for mortality and morbidity to the mother but also to her unborn child. Changes with pregnancy increase the risk of these patients to be a difficult airway. The best treatment for a difficult airway is a good assessment and preparation with backup plans available.

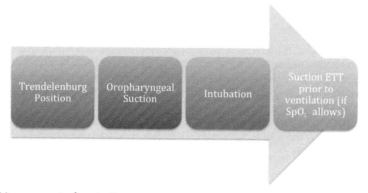

Fig. 2. Management of aspiration.

Risks of difficult airway

- Rapid desaturation of oxygen during apnea or hypoventilation due to
  o Increased oxygen consumption
  o Decreased functional residual capacity by 20% to 30%, cephalad displacement of diaphragm
  o Functional residual capacity (FRC) even closer to closing volume in patients with pre-existing lung disease, obesity, scoliosis, smoking, supine, or Trendelenburg position
  o Relative anemia of pregnancy

Patient evaluation (special consideration of)

- Increased edema of upper airway from an increase in extracellular fluid and decreased oncotic pressure
  o Worse with steep Trendelenburg or pre-eclampsia
- Friable mucosa, especially nasal mucosa due to capillary engorgement
- Enlarged breasts, which may impede laryngoscope handle positioning
- Increased Mallampati scores (**Fig. 3**)
- Full dentition

Planning for airway management
Proper positioning

1. Left uterine displacement to offload aortocaval compression
2. Sniffing position in nonobese
3. Ramped position (**Fig. 4**) with external auditory meatus and sternal notch aligned in a horizontal plane for obese patients

Have emergency airway equipment available:

1. Multiple laryngoscope blades/types (Macintosh 3, 4; Miller 2, 3)
2. Short laryngoscope handle (**Fig. 5**)
3. Several sizes of ETTs[6–8]
4. Oral and nasal airways
5. Stylet and bougie
6. Supraglottic device, laryngeal mask airway
7. Fiberoptic bronchoscope
8. Video laryngoscopy equipment
9. Availability of transtracheal jet ventilation or surgical airway (**Figs. 6** and **7**)

NEURAXIAL BLOCKADE
Introduction

Neuraxial blockade consists of either epidural or spinal blockade, the goal of which is to provide analgesia for delivery of the infant. For vaginal delivery, loss of pain sensation lower than T8 is the goal. Uterine contraction and cervical dilation result in visceral pain, which is transmitted at the T10 to L1 levels. As labor progresses and the fetal head descends, pressure on the pelvic floor, vagina, and perineum generate somatic pain transmitted by the pudendal nerve (S2–4). For cesarean delivery, a T4 level must be obtained (**Table 4**).

Hypotension

- Very common 30% to 40% of the time (**Fig. 8**)

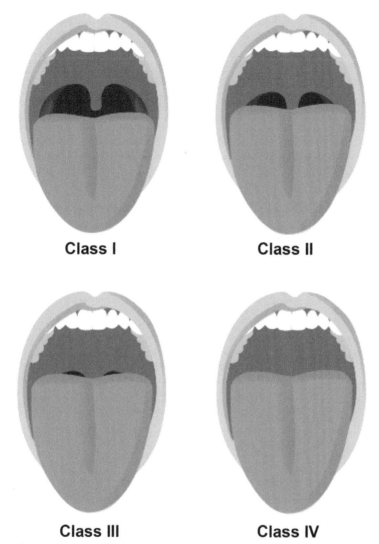

Fig. 3. Mallampati score. (*Courtesy of* Fotosearch. © Fotosearch.com; with permission.)

- Defined as systolic blood pressure less than 100 mm Hg or a 20% decrease from baseline[12]
- A large percentage of distress after epidural can be due to maternal hypotension
- Sympathetic efferents exit the spinal cord from T1 to L2[12,13]
- T1–T4 sympathectomy causes warm vasodilated hands, large reduction in systemic vascular resistance, and Horner syndrome and may lead to bradycardia due to blockade of cardiac accelerator fibers
- T5–L2 sympathectomy causes pooling of blood in the splanchnic vessels, reducing venous return and cardiac output[14]
- Inferior vena cava obstruction by gravid uterus further exacerbates a decrease in venous return[13]

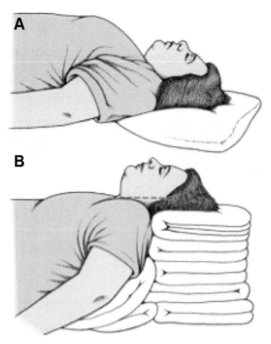

Fig. 4. Ramp position (*A*) Flat, no attempt at best airway position. (*B*) "Ear to sternal notch" position, or "ramped" position. (*Courtesy of* Fotosearch. © Fotosearch.com; with permission.)

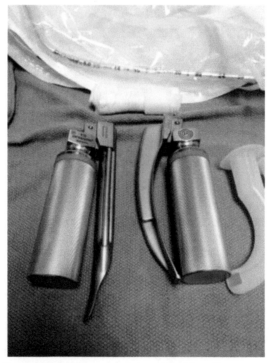

Fig. 5. Macintosh 3 and Miller 2 laryngoscopes on short handles.

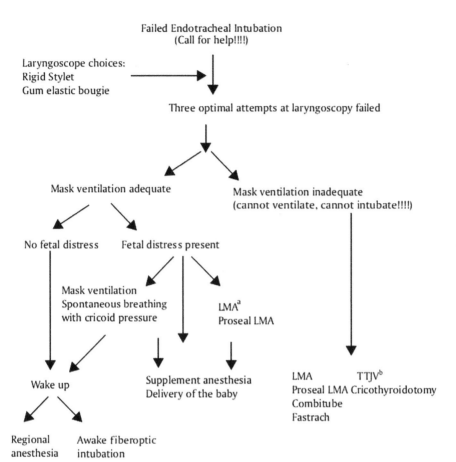

Fig. 6. Steps after trial of failed intubation during general anesthesia in obstetric patient.
[a] Laryngeal mask airway; [b] Transtracheal jet ventilation. (*From* Jadon A. Complications of regional and general anaesthesia in obstetric practice. Indian J Anaesth 2010;54(5):415–20.)

Patient evaluation overview
Monitor maternal blood pressure frequently after starting neuraxial blockade.

Summary/discussion
Maternal hypotension is a very common result of neuraxial anesthesia that should be anticipated and treated early. Before placement of a spinal or epidural block, consideration should be allowed for intravenous hydration to ensure the patient has adequate preload, which minimizes the effects of sympathectomy and vasodilation.

There is little downside to prophylactically treating small decreases in maternal blood pressure with vasoactive medications, expecting that left untreated, blood pressure will continue to decrease. The placenta does not have the ability to autoregulate; therefore, when maternal blood pressure is decreased, blood flow to the fetus is decreased, leading to fetal distress. Ensure that the mother is positioned such that the gravid uterus is not compressing the great vessels, optimize the fluid status in the mother, and treat with vasoactive medications as needed to restore maternal blood pressure normal levels (**Tables 5** and **6**).

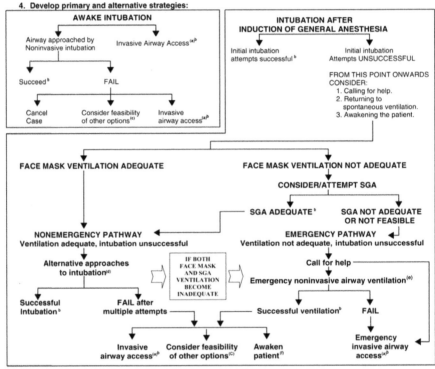

Fig. 7. ASA difficult airway algorithm. [a] Invasive airway access includes surgical or percutaneous airway, jet ventilation, and retrograde intubation. [b] Confirm ventilation, tracheal intubation, or SGA placement with exhaled CO_2. [c] Other options include (but are not limited to): surgery utilizing face mask or supraglottic airway (SGA) anesthesia (eg, LMA, ILMA, laryngeal tube), local anesthesia infiltration or regional nerve blockade. Pursuit of these options usually implies that mask ventilation will not be problematic. Therefore, these options may be of limited value if this step in the algorithm has been reached via the Emergency Pathway. [d] Alternative difficult intubation approaches include (but are not limited to): video-assisted laryngoscopy, alternative laryngoscope blades, SGA (eg, LMA or ILMA) as an intubation conduit (with or without fiberoptic guidance), fiberoptic intubation, intubating stylet or tube changer, light wand, and blind oral or nasal intubation. [e] Emergency non-invasive airway ventilation consists of a SGA. [f] Consider re-preparation of the patient for awake intubation or canceling surgery. (*From* Apfelbaum JL, Hagberg CA, Caplan RA, et al. Practice guidelines for management of the difficult airway: an updated report by the American Society of Anesthesiologists Task Force on Management of the Difficult Airway. Anesthesiology 2013;118(2):251–70; with permission.)

Table 4					
Common local anesthetics for spinal anesthesia					
			Duration (min)		
Drug	**Dose (mg) for T10**	**Dose (mg) for T4**	**Plain**	**+Epi**	**Onset (min)**
Lidocaine 5%	50–75	75–100	60–70	75–100	3–5
Bupivacaine 0.75%	8–12	14–20	90–110	100–150	5–8

Data from NYSORA. Spinal anesthesia. Available at: http://www.nysora.com/techniques/neuraxial-and-perineuraxial-techniques/landmark-based/3423-spinal-anesthesia.html.

High Spinal

- A respiratory and cardiac emergency
- Rapidly increasing sensory levels, dyspnea, bradycardia, apnea, and cardiac arrest after spinal or epidural bolus dose
- Most common with dosing an epidural that has unintentionally become intrathecal
- Occurs in ~1% of spinal anesthetics[15]
- Occurs when anesthetic level increases to higher than a T1 dermatome level (**Fig. 9**)

Patient evaluation overview

Hypotension[15]	Nausea
Bradycardia	Anxiety
Respiratory compromise	Cranial nerve involvement
Apnea	Arm/hand dyaesthesia or pain
Reduced oxygen saturation	Loss of consciousness
Difficulty speaking/coughing	Cardiac arrest (asystole)

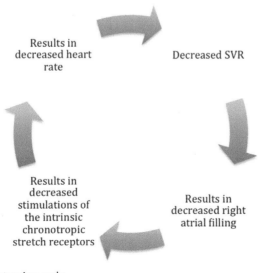

Results in decreased heart rate

Decreased SVR

Results in decreased right atrial filling

Results in decreased stimulations of the intrinsic chronotropic stretch receptors

Fig. 8. Spinal hypotension cycle.

Table 5
Pharmacologic treatment options

Intravenous Fluid (IVF)	500 mL to 1 L rapid bolus. Preload with 1 L IVF before blockade
Phenylephrine	100 µg IV, repeat as needed (may lead to reflex bradycardia)
Ephedrine	5–10 mg IV, repeat as needed (may lead to tachyphylaxis)

Data from Pellegrini JE. Prevention and treatment of spinal induced hypotension. Available at: http://www.aana.com/meetings/meeting-materials/annualcongress/Documents/Pellegrini_Handouts.pdf.

Combination therapies

1. Notify attending anesthesiologist
   a. Consider calling a STAT
2. Inform obstetrician or surgeon
3. Support ventilation and intubate if necessary
4. Support blood pressure with intravenous (IV) fluid bolus and vasopressors (**Table 7**)
5. Treat bradycardia with epinephrine (preferred to atropine)
6. Consider:
   a. Emergency cesarean section if signs of fetal distress
   b. Need for more venous access
   c. Sedation until able to extubate (midazolam)
   d. Treat cardiac arrest with advanced cardiac life support (ACLS) protocols

Causes

- Excessive dose of local anesthetic
- Failure to reduce normally accepted dose in patients susceptible to excessive spread (pregnant, obese, or short patients)
- Unusual excessive spread
- Spinal anesthetic after recent epidural bolus dose[16]

Table 6
Nonpharmacologic treatment options

Oxygen	If there is fetal bradycardia
Reposition	Left uterine displacement, hands and knees, etc

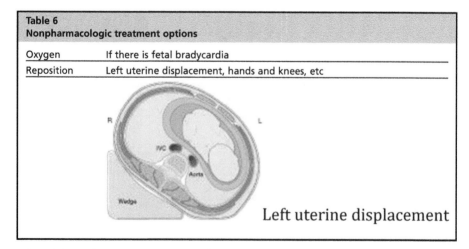

Left uterine displacement

Adapted from Pellegrini JE. Prevention and treatment of spinal induced hypotension. Available at: http://www.aana.com/meetings/meeting-materials/annualcongress/Documents/Pellegrini_Handouts.pdf; with permission.

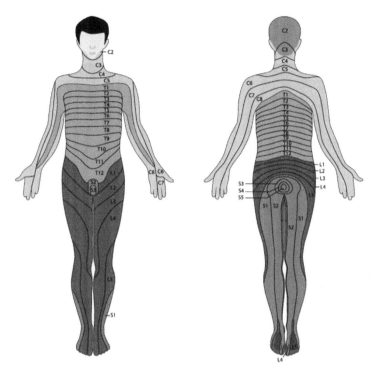

Fig. 9. Dermatome Map. (*Courtesy of* Fotosearch. © Fotosearch.com; with permission.)

Summary/discussion

High or total spinal blockade occurs when spinal blockade increase to higher than the T1 dermatomal level and can lead to cardiovascular collapse and respiratory arrest. Symptoms and signs of high spinal usually occur within minutes of placement; however, delay of up to 30 minutes has been reported.[15] Nausea and anxiety, both from cerebral hypoperfusion, are usually the first reported symptoms.

Prevention of high spinal anesthesia, while not always possible, is based on frequent monitoring of sensory levels, patient positioning to influence spread of medication via baricity, and recognition for timely intervention in the event of circulatory collapse.

Local Anesthetic Systemic Toxicity

Table 8

- Local anesthetics act on sodium channels, and therefore, local anesthetic systemic toxicity (LAST) is seen in organs of the body that depend on these sodium

Table 7 Pharmacologic treatment options	
Epinephrine	5–10 µg IV bolus dosing
Vasopressin	1–2 units IV bolus dosing
Atropine	0.5–1 mg IV bolus

Table 8 Local anesthetic maximum doses (mg/kg)		
	Plain	+ Epi
Lidocaine	5	7
Mepivacaine	5	7 (400 mg max)
Bupivacaine/Ropivacaine	3	3

Data from Open Anesthesia. Local anesthetics: systemic toxicity. Available at https://www.openanesthesia.org/local_anesthetics_systemic_toxicity/.

channels for proper function, such as the central nervous system (CNS) and the heart.
- The CNS is more sensitive to the effects of local anesthetics than the cardiac system and will generally manifest symptoms of toxicity first.

Signs/symptoms
Table 9

Combination therapies

1. Notify attending anesthesiologist[17]
   a. Consider calling a STAT
2. Notify surgical team (if in operating room)
3. Change Fio_2 to 100% (avoid hypoxia) and hyperventilate (avoid acidosis). Intubate if not already done.
4. Treat seizures with benzodiazepines.
5. Call for lipid emulsion and cardiac bypass (if cardiotoxicity).
6. Administer lipid emulsion 20% (DO NOT USE propofol; it is only 10% and is likely to lead to severe hypotension).
7. Start a second IV.
8. Consider ACLS modifications:
   a. Administer low-dose epinephrine, 1 μg/kg IV
   b. Avoid vasopressin (can cause pulmonary edema)
9. Consider:
   a. Monitor patient postoperatively in intensive care unit.
   b. Perform cardiopulmonary bypass if refractory cardiac arrest (STAT page perfusion for setup) (**Fig. 10**).

Table 9 Signs and Symptoms of Local Anesthesitc Toxicity (LAST)			
Central Nervous System			Cardiac
Excitation	Depression	Nonspecific	—
Agitation	Drowsiness	Diplopia	Hypotension
Tremors	Coma	Dizziness	Bradycardia
Seizure	Slurred speech	—	Asystole
Metallic taste	—	—	Atrial/ventricular ectopy
Circumoral numbness	—	—	—
Tinnitus	—	—	—

Data from Neal JM, Bernards CM, Butterworth JM, et al. ASRA practice advisory of local anesthetic systemic toxicity. Reg Anesth Pain Med 2010;35(2):152–61; and Checklist for treatment of local anesthetic systemic toxicity. ASRA.

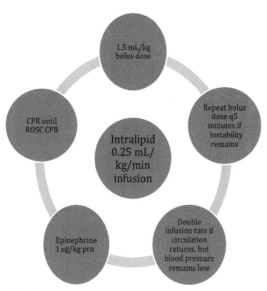

Fig. 10. Treatment of LAST.

Summary/discussion
Local anesthetic systemic toxicity is a rare but serious complication of obstetric anesthesia. Rapid recognition and early treatment with intralipid are key to good outcomes.

Persistent Neuropathy

- Neurologic injury after labor and delivery may be intrinsic to the labor/delivery process or may result directory or indirectly from obstetric of anesthetic intervention.[18]
- Sixteen percent of obstetric claims in the ASA's Closed Claims Database were for maternal nerve damage.[19]
- Acute injury to nerves can occur by several mechanisms:
  - Direct trauma to nerve tissue from nerve transection, stretch, or compression
  - Nerve trauma from needles or catheters
  - Intraneuronal injection of anesthetic agents or other toxins
  - Ischemia from trauma, compression, or stretch injuries to supporting vascular structures
- Neuropathy refers to damage to a peripheral nerve regardless of the cause.
- Recovery of nerve function after injury is predicted by the percentage of axonal loss with an axonal loss less than 50% predicting recovery within 1 year (**Fig. 11**).

Avoidance of direct trauma during neuraxial anesthesia
The spinal cord terminates into the cauda equina at the L1 vertebral body in most adults. Neuraxial should be performed lower than L3 as estimated by the anesthesiologist, based on anatomic landmarks. In addition, it is recommended to halt needle advancement immediately if the parturient perceives pain, especially if there is pain during injection of anesthetic solution. If the pain recurs on initiation of injection, the needle/catheter should be repositioned, and if still painful, it should be removed. A transient parasthesia is not uncommon during placement of a catheter.

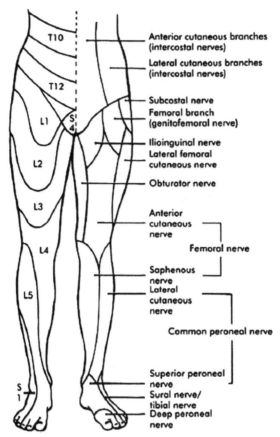

Anterior cutaneous branches
(intercostal nerves)

Lateral cutaneous branches
(intercostal nerves)

Subcostal nerve
Femoral branch
(genitofemoral nerve)

Ilioinguinal nerve
Lateral femoral
cutaneous nerve

Obturator nerve

Anterior
cutaneous
nerve

Femoral nerve

Saphenous
nerve
Lateral
cutaneous
nerve

Common peroneal nerve

Superior peroneal
nerve
Sural nerve/
tibial nerve
Deep peroneal
nerve

T10
T12
L1
L2
L3
L4
L5
S1
S4

Avoidance of Direct Trauma During Neuraxial Anesthesia

Fig. 11. Innervation of the lower extremity. (*From* Haymaker W, Woodhall B. Peripheral nerve injuries, 2d ed. Philadelphia: Saunders; 1953.)

Evaluation overview

Initial evaluation of the patient should include the presence of lower extremity pain, numbness, or weakness (**Table 10**). This information should be used in the risk/benefit discussion when discussing neuraxial anesthesia with the parturient (**Fig. 12**).

Evaluation of postpartum complaints of lower extremity numbness, weakness, and pain should occur promptly, and rare life- or limb-threatening causes should be ruled out. Symptoms present immediately after delivery, and those that have improved or stayed the same, are less likely to be more life-threatening than those that occur suddenly and after a symptom-free period. A complete history and physical examination should include determination of the onset time of symptoms and details of the labor and delivery process (eg, mode of delivery, use of forceps, maternal positioning).

The presence of a fever and elevated white blood count suggest the presence of infection, whereas sensory and motor deficits without pain suggest an intrinsic obstetric palsy (see **Table 10**). A detailed neurologic examination will help in differentiation between central, radicular, plexus, and peripheral nerve lesions may be considered. More complex symptoms, particularly motor deficits, or bilateral symptoms, should

Table 10
Obstetric Palsies

Palsy	Cause/Risks	Symptoms
Lateral femoral cutaneous	Trauma, prolonged hip flexion, exaggerated lumbar lordosis	Loss of sensation to the lateral thigh
Femoral	Pfannenstiel incision, self-retaining retractors, thigh flexion with external rotation and abduction	Weakness of hip flexion, loss of sensation medial lower leg
Lumbosacral plexus	Compression by fetal head against the pelvis, forceps delivery	Foot drop (**Table 11**)
Peroneal	External compression from pressure at the head of the fibula, usually from stirrups	Numbness of the lateral leg and dorsum of the foot, weakness of foot dorsiflexion, and eversion
Sciatic	Stretch, injection trauma	Weakness of foot inversion, absent ankle jerk

prompt consultation with a neurologist or neurosurgeon. Immediate MRI is the current gold standard to rule out central lesions. Electromyography (EMG) may aid in determining the site of injury as well as the degree of axonal loss; however, EMG only measures large nerve fiber changes and may take as long as 3 weeks after injury to show changes. An abnormal EMG in the first postpartum week suggests pre-existing injury.[18,19]

Table 11
Differential diagnosis of foot drop

	L5 Nerve Root	Lumbar Plexus	Sciatic Nerve	Peroneal Nerve
Motor	Weakness of paraspinous muscles	Weakness of gluteal muscles and anal sphincter	—	—
Ankle inversion[a]	Weak	Weak	Normal or weak	Normal
Plantar flexion	Normal	Normal	Normal or weak	Normal
Toe flexion	Weak	Weak	Normal or weak	Normal
Sensory loss	Poorly demarcated, predominately big toe	Well demarcated to L5 dermatome	Lower 2/3 of lateral leg, and dorsum of foot	Lower 2/3 of lateral leg and dorsum of foot
Ankle jerk	Normal[b]	Normal[b]	Normal or weak	Normal
Pain	Common, radicular	Common, may be radicular	Can be severe	Rare

[a] Attempt at inversion should be made with the foot dorsiflexed passively to 90°.
[b] Weak with S1 involvement.
From Katirji B. Entrapment and other focal neuropathies. Peroneal Neuropathy. Neurol Clin 1999;17:567–91; with permission.

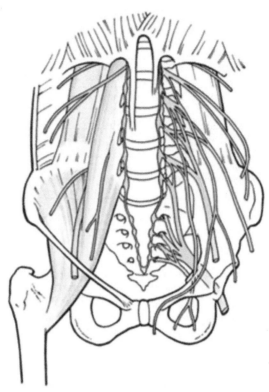

Fig. 12. Innervation of the pelvic outlet.

Transient Neurologic Symptoms

- Transient neurologic symptoms (TNS) is a painful condition of the buttocks and thighs with possible radiation to the lower extremities.[20]
- Symptoms may start a few hours after a spinal anesthetic and may last as long as 10 days.
- Incidence is 1 in 7 with intrathecal lidocaine/Mepivacaine (7-fold less incidence for intrathecal bupivacaine).
- Differentiated from cauda quina syndrome, as TNS is exclusively a pain syndrome: there is no associated muscle weakness or loss of bowel or bladder function.
- Treatment is reassurance and monitoring with the expectation that symptoms will resolve within 10 days.[21]
- Early ambulation seems to help with resolution of symptoms (**Box 1**).

Postdural Puncture Headache

- Positional headache: Exacerbated by sitting or standing and alleviated by lying flat (**Fig. 13**)
- Caused by dural puncture which results in leakage of cerebral spinal fluid (CSF), which leads to intracranial hypotension and reduction of CSF volume
  - Decreased cushioning of the brain
  - Traction placed on the brain while in the upright position
  - Vasodilation as the body attempts to replace CSF that is leaking through the dural puncture

Box 1
Risk factors for transient neurologic symptoms
5% Lidocaine
Lithotomy position
Microcatheter use
Outpatient status
Data from Sime AC. AANA Journal course: transient neurological symptoms and spinal anesthesia. AANA J 2000;68:163–827.

- Expected rate of dural puncture (wet tap) with lumbar epidural is ~1.5%.[22]
  - Independent of performer skill or expertise
  - Risk of developing postdural puncture headache (PDPH) as a result of a wet tap is ~52% (**Table 12**)
- PDPH from spinal anesthesia is related to the gauge and shape of the needle used, with smaller-gauge pencil-point needles having the lowest incidence of PDPH (**Fig. 14**).
  - In the picture on the left in **Fig. 14**, Whitacre and Sprote are examples of pencil-point needles.
  - The Quincke has a cutting tip and is associated with a higher incidence of PDPH.

Differential diagnosis of postpartum headache

- Lactation headache[23]
- Migraine
- Subdural hematoma
- Brain mass/tumor
- Arterial venous malformation
- Cortical vein/dural sinus thrombosis
- Tension headache
- Pre-eclampsia
- Pneumocephalus
- Dehydration

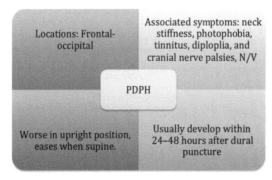

Fig. 13. PDPH signs and symptoms.

Table 12 Risk factors for dural puncture and PDPH	
Risk Factors for Dural Puncture	**Risk Factors for PDPH**
Increased body mass index	Low body mass index
Increased age	Pregnancy
	Prior history of PDPH
	Younger age[a]
	Needle gauge/type

[a] Elderly patients will have reduced elasticity of the dura mater, which increases the resistance to CSF leakage.

- Caffeine withdrawal
- Meningitis/encephalitis

Treatment options
Treatment options for PDPH are outlined in **Fig. 15**.

Epidural blood patch
Epidural blood patching (EBP) involves the injection of autologous blood into the epidural space.

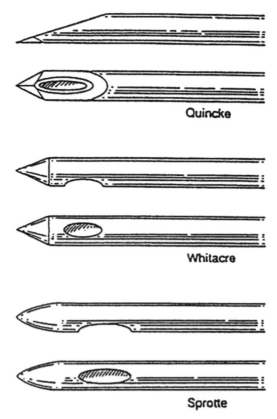

Quincke

Whitacre

Sprotte

Fig. 14. Spinal needles. (*From* Peterman SB. Postmyelography headache rates with Whitacre versus Quincke 22-gauge spinal needles. Radiology 1996;200:771–8; with permission.)

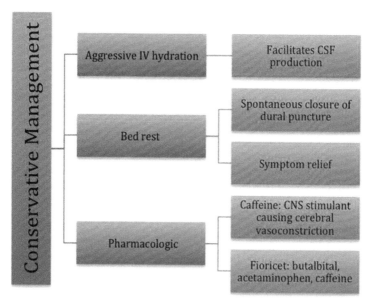

Fig. 15. Treatment of PDPH.

The exact mechanism of action is unknown; however, the leading hypothesis is that the resulting blood clot may have a "patch effect" on the dural tear, while the volume of blood transfused into the epidural space raises intracranial pressure and reduces ongoing CSF leak.[24]

- Considered definitive treatment of PDPH
- Efficacy is ~90% for first blood patch
- If second blood patch is required, efficacy is ~97%
- Contraindications to EBP include sepsis, leukocytosis, fever, coagulopathy, and patient refusal
- Risks of EBP include those of epidural placement (bleeding, infection, PDPH, nerve injury) as well as meningitis, arachnoiditis, and cauda equine syndrome.
- EBP should be performed by 2 clinicians.
  - One clinician should be trained in neuraxial technics (an anesthesiologist)
  - The second clinician will need to draw a volume of blood from the patient's arm via a new venous stick
  - Both should use full aseptic technique
- 12 to 20 mL of autologous blood is injected into the epidural space
- Patient should experience almost immediate headache relief
- The patient should lie flat for 1 to 2 hours after EBP to allow time for the blood to coagulate

OBSTETRIC LIFE SUPPORT

As part of the Stanford anesthesia informatics and media laboratory project, a cognitive aid for treatment of maternal arrest was released in February 2013.[25] It is available for view at: http://www.anesthesiaillustrated.org/cogaids/obstetric-cardiac-arrest-aids/, and the download was done in compliance with creative commons attribution-noncommercial-noderivs 3.0 unported licenses (Appendix 1).

REFERENCES

1. Kreppel D, Antoniadis G, Seeling W. Spinal hematoma: a literature survey with meta-analysis of 613 patients. Neurosurg Rev 2003;26:1–49.
2. Levine MN, Raskob G, Landefelt S, et al. Hemorrhagic complications of anti-coagulant treatment. Chest 2001;110:108S–21S.
3. Vandermeulen EP, Van Aken H, Vermylen J, et al. Anticoagulants and spinal-epidural anesthesia. Anesth Analg 1994;79:1165–77.
4. Available at: https://www.asra.com/advisory-guidelines/article/1/anticoagulation-3rd-edition.
5. Available at: http://www.asahq.org/~/media/Sites/ASAHQ/Files/Public/Resources/standards-guidelines/guidelines-for-neuraxial-anesthesia-in-obstetrics.pdf.
6. Available at: http://anes.med.umich.edu/vault/1007575-AnticoagulationNeuraxial Guidelines.pdf.
7. Lawton MT, Porter RW, Heiserman JE, et al. Surgical management of spinal epidural hematoma: relationship between surgical timing and neurological outcome. J Neurosurg 1995;83(1):1–7.
8. Kodali B, Chandrasekhar S, Bulich LN. Airway changes during labor and delivery. Anesthesiology 2008;108:357–62.
9. American Society of Anesthesiologists Committee. Practice guidelines for preoperative fasting and the use of pharmacologic agents to reduce the risk of pulmonary aspiration: application to healthy patients undergoing elective procedures. An updated report by the American Society of Anesthesiologists Committee on Standards and Practice Parameters. Anesthesiology 2011;114(3):495–511.
10. Marik PE. Aspiration pneumonitis and aspiration pneumonia. N Engl J Med 2001;344(9):665–71.
11. Hawkins JL, Chang J, Palmer SK, et al. Anesthesia-related maternal mortality in the United States. 1979-2002. Obstet Gynecol 2011;117(1):69–74.
12. Kiohr S, Roth R, Hormann T, et al. Definitions of hypotension after spinal anaesthesia for caesarean section: literature search and application to parturients. Acta Anaesthesiol Scand 2010;54(8):909–21.
13. Clark RB. Hypotension and caesarean section. Br J Anaesth 2008;101(6):882.
14. NYSORA. Spinal anesthesia. Available at: http://www.nysora.com/techniques/neuraxial-and-perineuraxial-techniques/landmark-based/3423-spinal-anesthesia.html.
15. Neuman B. Complete spinal block following spinal anaesthesia. Anaesthesia tutorial of the week. 24th May 2010.
16. Furst SR, Reisner LS. Risk of high spinal anesthesia following failed epidural block for cesarean delivery. J Clin Anesth 1995;7(1):71–4.
17. Checklist for treatment of local anesthetic systemic toxicity. ASRA.
18. Cynthia Wong. Neurologic Deficit and Labor Analgesia.
19. ASA Closed Claims Project.
20. Open Anesthesia. Local Anesthetics: Transient Neurologic Symptoms.
21. Sime AC. AANA journal course: transient neurological symptoms and spinal anesthesia. AANA J 2000;68:163–8.
22. Choi PT, Galinski SE, Takeuchi L, et al. PDPH is a common complication of neuraxial blockade in parturients: a meta-analysis of obstetrical studies. Can J Anaesth 2003;50(5):406–9.

23. Jadon A. Complications of regional and general anaesthesia in obstetric practice. Indian J Anaesth 2010;54(5):415–20.
24. Jane Campbell FRCA. Effective management of the post-dural puncture headache. Anesthesia tutorial of the week. 31st May 2010.
25. Chu L, Harrison K. CogAIDs Project, Stanford AIM Lab (Anesthesia Informatics and Media Lab. Anesthesiaillustrated.org).

APPENDIX 1: Obstetric life support cognitive aide. *From* Anesthesia Informatics and Media Lab, Stanford, CA. Designed by Larry Chu, MD. Available at: http://aim.stanford.edu/project/anesthesiaillustrated/.

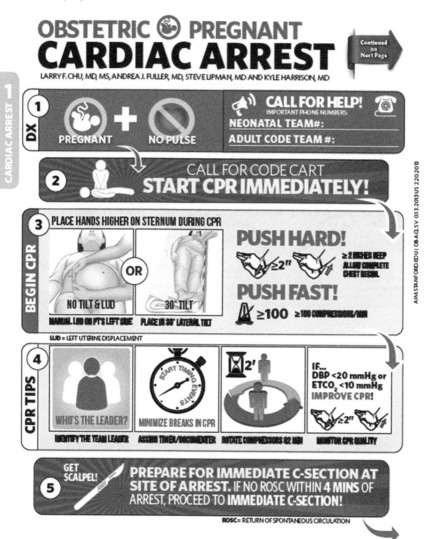

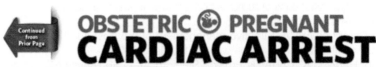

OBSTETRIC PREGNANT
CARDIAC ARREST

LARRY F. CHU, MD, MS, ANDREA J. FULLER, MD, STEVE LIPMAN, MD AND KYLE HARRISON, MD

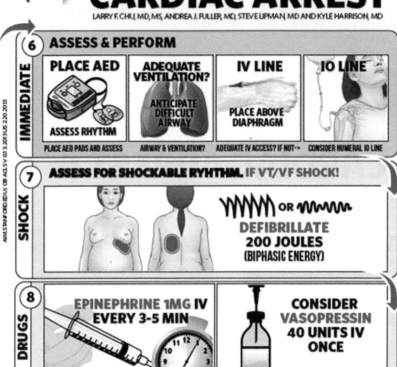

6 ASSESS & PERFORM

IMMEDIATE

PLACE AED	ADEQUATE VENTILATION?	IV LINE	IO LINE
ASSESS RHYTHM	ANTICIPATE DIFFICULT AIRWAY	PLACE ABOVE DIAPHRAGM	
PLACE AED PADS AND ASSESS	AIRWAY & VENTILATION?	ADEQUATE IV ACCESS? IF NOT->	CONSIDER HUMERAL IO LINE

7 ASSESS FOR SHOCKABLE RYHTHM. IF VT/VF SHOCK!

SHOCK

OR

DEFIBRILLATE
200 JOULES
(BIPHASIC ENERGY)

8 DRUGS

EPINEPHRINE 1MG IV EVERY 3-5 MIN	CONSIDER VASOPRESSIN 40 UNITS IV ONCE
IF POSSIBLE ASSIGN PERSON TO TIME & ADMINISTER DOSES	VASOPRESSIN DOSE COULD REPLACE ONE EPINEPHRINE DOSE

CARDIAC ARREST   1

Reference: 1) Part 12: Cardiac Arrest in Special Situations : 2010 American Heart Association Guidelines for Cardiopulmonary Resuscitation and Emergency Cardiovascular Care. Vanden Hoek et al, Circulation. 2010;122:S829-S861. 2) Maternal CPR Illustrations by Ms. Janet Fong. WWW.AIC.CUHK.EDU.HK/WEB8

Continued from Prior Page

OBSTETRIC 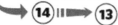 PREGNANT
CARDIAC ARREST

LARRY F. CHU, MD, MS, ANDREA J. FULLER, MD, STEVE LIPMAN, MD AND KYLE HARRISON, MD

CARDIAC ARREST 1

CONT. CPR 9

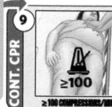

≥100

≥100 COMPRESSIONS/MIN

MINIMIZE BREAKS IN CPR

 2'

ROTATE COMPRESSORS Q2 MIN

IF...
DBP <20 mmHg or
$ETCO_2$ <10 mmHg
IMPROVE CPR!

≥2"

MONITOR CPR QUALITY

AIM.STANFORD.EDU | OB.ACLS.V 013.2013.US 22O.2013

TX 10

REPEAT CYCLE UNTIL RESUSCITATED
CPR + DEFIBRILLATE (IF VT/VF) EVERY 2 MINS + DRUGS

OTHER 11

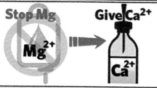

Stop Mg   Give Ca^{2+}

Mg^{2+} Ca^{2+}

IF RUNNING, STOP MAG INFUSION, GIVE 10% CACL₂ 10CC IV

10/min

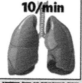

VENTILATE 10 BREATHS/MIN

100% O_2

DELIVER 100% OXYGEN

R/O CAUSES 12

FIRST RULE OUT COMMON TREATABLE CAUSES

PEA/ASYSTOLE	VF/VT	OTHER CAUSES
1) Bleeding	1) Hyperkalemia	CONTINUE TO #13 TO RULE OUT
2) Drug Toxicity	2) Coronary Thrombosis	OTHER CAUSES & TREATMENT
LOCAL ANESTHETIC, MG, OXYTOCIN	3) HypoMg or Torsades	GUIDELINES.
3) High Spinal		
4) Hypoventilation	TX: Consider Antiarrythmics	CONTINUE TO #14 FOR VF/VT
5) Embolism	AMIODARONE 300 MG IV OR	TREATMENT GUIDELINES
PULMONARY, AFE, VAE	LIDOCAINE 100 MG IV	

13   14 || 13

Continued on Next Page

OBSTETRIC
CARDIAC ARREST

LARRY F. CHU, MD, MS, ANDREA J. FULLER, MD, STEVE LIPMAN, MD AND KYLE HARRISON, MD

CARDIAC ARREST **1**

FIND TREATABLE CAUSES – BEAU-CHOPS

AIMS.STANFORD.EDU | 08 AXLS V 03.1.2013 | US 2.20.2013

(13) CROSS-CHECK POSSIBLE CAUSES WITH TEAM FOR DIAGNOSIS

BLEEDING/DIC

IF SUSPECTED THEN:
1) Rapid bolus IV Fluids.
2) Activate MTG.
3) Consider transfusion of blood products.
4) Consider placement of arterial line.

EMBOLISM
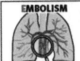

IF PULMONARY EMBOLISM:
1) Consider TEE/TTE to rule out RV failure.
2) Consider thrombolytic therapy– discuss risk/ benefits with team.

ANESTHETICS

ANESTHETIC COMPLICATIONS INCLUDE:
1) Spinal shock from regional anesthesia
2) Local anesthetic toxicity
3) Loss of airway or ventilation

UTERINE ATONY

IF SUSPECTED CONSIDER:
1) Oxytocin
2) Misoprostol
3) Methylergonovine
4) Carboprost
5) Bimanual fundal massage

CARDIAC DISEASE

IF SUSPECTED CONSIDER:
1) Myocardial infarction – consider percutaneous coronary intervention.
2) Aortic dissection
   - Consider cardiac surgery consult
3) Congenital heart disease
   - Consider cards consult
4) Pulmonary hypertension
   - Consider NO.
5) Magnesium toxicity
   - Consider CaC1, 1gm IV

HYPERTENSION

IF SUSPECTED CONSIDER:
1) Pre-eclampsia
2) Eclampsia

PLACENTA

IF SUSPECTED CONSIDER:
1) Placenta abruptio
2) Placenta accreta

SEPSIS

IF SUSPECTED CONSIDER:
1) Goals: CVP ≥8-12mmHg, MAP≥65mmHg, Urine output≥0.5ml/kg/h, MVO, Sat≥65%.
2) Fluid therapy
3) Antimicrobial therapy
4) Removing source of sepsis

Continued from Prior Page

Continued on Next Page

OBSTETRIC PREGNANT
CARDIAC ARREST

LARRY F. CHU, MD, MS, ANDREA J. FULLER, MD, STEVE LIPMAN, MD AND KYLE HARRISON, MD

CARDIAC ARREST 1

FIND TREATABLE CAUSES - BEAU-CHOPS

(13) CROSS-CHECK POSSIBLE CAUSES WITH TEAM FOR DIAGNOSIS

PNEUMOTHORAX

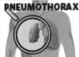

SUSPECT IF:
Unilateral breath sounds, ↑ neck veins, ⇨ trachea

IF SUSPECTED:
Perform **needle decompression** (Midclavicular line 2nd intercostal space) **and chest tube.**

ABG TO RULE OUT

RULE OUT:
1) Hyperkalemia
2) Hypocalcemia
3) Acidosis
4) Hypoglycemia
5) Hypokalemia

CORONARY THROMBOSIS

IF SUSPECTED THEN:
1) Consider TEE
2) Consider emergent revascularization or cath lab.
3) Consider intra aortic balloon pump

HYPOXIA

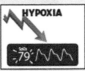

IF SUSPECTED THEN:
1) 100% FiO₂. In OR: rule out switched gas lines. Use separate O₂ tank.
2) Check connections Re-confirm ET tube placement.
3) Confirm bilateral breath sounds.
4) Suction ET tube.
5) Rule out other causes with TTE/TEE.

CARDIAC TAMPONADE

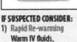

SUSPECT IF:
1) ↑ CVP, equalization of right & left- sided pressures.
2) Consider TEE/TTE to rule out pericardial effusion.
3) If present, perform pericardiocentisis.

HYPO/HYPERTHERMIA

IF SUSPECTED CONSIDER:
1) Rapid Re-warming Warm IV fluids, peritoneal lavage, ECMO or CPB

IF >40°C THEN:
1) Rule out malignant hyperthermia and treat if found.

TOXINS

CONSIDER ALL MEDS RECEIVED INCLUDING:
1) Existing infusions
2) Prescribed medications
3) Illicit drug use
4) Syringe swaps or drug errors
5) Poisoning

IF SUSPECTED THEN:
1) Contact poison control/ pharmacy
2) Administer appropriate therapy/antidote

POISON

FOR A POISON EMERGENCY IN THE UNITED STATES:
1) Call 1-800-222-1222

Continued on Next Page

Continued from Prior Page

Continued from Prior Page

OBSTETRIC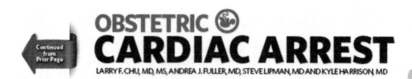
CARDIAC ARREST

LARRY F. CHU, MD, MS, ANDREA J. FULLER, MD, STEVE LIPMAN, MD AND KYLE HARRISON, MD

AIMS.STANFORD.EDU | OB A/CL S V 0.1 3.2013/US 2.20.2013

VT/VFIB CONSIDERATIONS

(14)

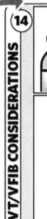

CONSIDER ANTIARRYTHMICS

AMIODARONE 300 MG IV OR
LIDOCAINE 100 MG IV

CORONARY THROMBOSIS?

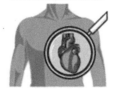

IF SUSPECTED THEN:

1) CONSIDER TTE.
2) CONSIDER EMERGENT REVASCULARIZATION/CATH LAB.
3) CONSIDER INTRA AORTIC BALLOON PUMP.

HYPERKALEMIA?

CHECK A BG:

>7.0 MMOL/L
LIFE THREATENING

6.1-6.9 MMOL/L
MODERATE

CONSIDER: INSULIN 10 UNITS IV WITH GLUCOSE 40-60GM IV[1]

CONSIDER:
20 ML 10% CALCIUM-GLUCONATE IV
(OVER 5-10 MIN*, REPEAT IF NEEDED)[2]

ALSO CONSIDER: SALBUMETOL 0.5 MG IV[1]

IF PH<7.20 CONSIDER:
BICARBONATE 1-2 AMPS IV[1]

*INFUSE OVER 20-30 MIN IF PATIENT ON DIGOXIN

↓MG OR TORSADES?

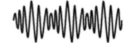

CONSIDER MgSO₄ 2GM IV

[1] Ahee P. and Crowe A.V. The management of hyperkalemia in the emergency department. J Accid Emerg Med 2000;17:188-191
[2] Allon M. Treatment and prevention of hyperkalemia in end-stage renal disease. Kidney Int. 1993;43:1197-209.

CARDIAC ARREST 1

Hypertensive Emergencies in Pregnancy

Courtney Olson-Chen, MD, Neil S. Seligman, MD, MS*

KEYWORDS

- Hypertensive disorders • Pregnancy • Gestational hypertension • Preeclampsia
- Antihypertensive medications

KEY POINTS

- The 4 main categories of hypertensive disorders in pregnancy are chronic hypertension, gestational hypertension, preeclampsia, and chronic hypertension with superimposed preeclampsia.
- Hypertensive disorders contribute to significant maternal, fetal, and neonatal morbidity and mortality.
- The pathophysiology and etiology of hypertensive disorders in pregnancy is not well understood.
- All antihypertensive drugs cross the placenta, and only a few medications have been sufficiently studied in pregnancy.
- Untreated severe maternal hypertension can lead to end-organ injury. First-line medications for severe hypertension include intravenous labetalol, intravenous hydralazine, and oral nifedipine.

INTRODUCTION

Classification of Hypertensive Disorders in Pregnancy

There are 4 categories of hypertensive disorders in pregnancy as outlined by the 2013 American College of Obstetricians and Gynecologists (ACOG) Task Force on Hypertension in Pregnancy.[1] This group of experts was convened to review available data and provide evidence-based guidelines for the diagnosis and management of hypertensive disorders in pregnancy. The 4 categories include chronic hypertension (CHTN), preeclampsia, gestational hypertension (GHTN), and CHTN with superimposed preeclampsia.

Disclosure Statement: Neither of the authors have any commercial or financial conflicts of interest to declare. No funding was received for this article.
Division of Maternal-Fetal Medicine, Department of Obstetrics and Gynecology, University of Rochester Medical Center, 601 Elmwood Avenue, Box 668, Rochester, NY 14642, USA
* Corresponding author.
E-mail address: Neil_Seligman@urmc.rochester.edu

Crit Care Clin 32 (2016) 29–41
http://dx.doi.org/10.1016/j.ccc.2015.08.006
criticalcare.theclinics.com
0749-0704/16/$ – see front matter © 2016 Elsevier Inc. All rights reserved.

CHTN is an increase in blood pressure that either antedates pregnancy or begins before 20 weeks of gestation. Preeclampsia involves an elevation in blood pressure after 20 weeks of gestation in addition to either proteinuria or the development of signs of end-organ damage known as "severe features" (**Box 1**). Proteinuria is defined as excretion of 300 mg or greater of protein in a 24-h urine collection or a random protein to creatinine ratio of at least 0.3 mg/dL. Importantly, the ACOG recently emphasized that proteinuria is not requisite for the diagnosis of preeclampsia.[1] Preeclampsia can be subdivided into preeclampsia and preeclampsia with severe features based on the presence of severely elevated blood pressure or the aforementioned severe signs and symptoms.[2] The amount of protein is no longer used to differentiate preeclampsia and preeclampsia with severe features. GHTN occurs when there is an increase in blood pressure after 20 weeks of gestation in the absence of proteinuria or other severe features of preeclampsia. Finally, preeclampsia can occur in patients with longstanding CHTN. This category is referred to as CHTN with superimposed preeclampsia.[1]

A non–pregnancy-related acute increase in blood pressure known as a "hypertensive emergency" may also occur in pregnant patients. This life-threatening presentation necessitates immediate treatment. Examples of this clinical scenario include hypertensive encephalopathy, aortic dissection, left ventricular failure, and increased catecholamines secondary to conditions such as pheochromocytoma or cocaine intoxication.[3] Some of these diagnoses, like hypertensive encephalopathy, can be difficult to differentiate from preeclampsia. A retrospective study found that hypertensive encephalopathy is quite rare in comparison with preeclampsia.[4]

Epidemiology of Hypertensive Disorders in Pregnancy

An increasing number of pregnant women in the United States have chronic medical conditions, like CHTN, that increase the risk of adverse outcomes.[5] The prevalence of hypertensive disorders in pregnancy has been increasing over the last decade with up to 8% of deliveries affected in 2006.[6] A cross-sectional study of national data found that the increased prevalence of hypertensive disorders was highest for CHTN and GHTN, but rates of preeclampsia are also increasing.[6] In fact, since 1987, the incidence of preeclampsia has increased by approximately 25% in the United States.[7] Hypertensive disorders are more common in women with multiple gestations, chronic medical conditions, and gestational diabetes.[6] The prevalence of hypertension is expected to continue to increase in the future with advancing maternal age and rising rates of obesity.[8]

Hypertensive disorders are a predominant cause of maternal and perinatal morbidity and mortality around the world.[2] From 2006 to 2010, hypertensive disorders

---

Box 1
Severe features of preeclampsia

- Severe hypertension (systolic BP $\geq$160 mm Hg or diastolic BP $\geq$110 mm Hg)
- Thrombocytopenia (platelets <100,000/μL)
- Elevated liver enzymes (twice normal)
- Right upper quadrant or epigastric pain unresponsive to medication
- Unremitting cerebral or visual symptoms
- Renal insufficiency (creatinine >1.1 mg/dL or twice normal)
- Pulmonary edema

Abbreviation: BP, blood pressure.

accounted for 9.4% of pregnancy-related deaths in the United States.[5] The majority of maternal deaths related to hypertensive disorders of pregnancy occur within 42 days postpartum. Severe maternal complications occurring significantly more often in women with hypertensive disorders compared with normotensive women include acute renal failure, disseminated intravascular coagulation syndrome, pulmonary edema, pulmonary embolism, cerebrovascular disorders, and respiratory distress. Severe obstetric complications are most likely to occur in preeclampsia with severe features but also occur in GHTN, although the risk is comparatively modest.[6] Adverse fetal and neonatal outcomes, including iatrogenic preterm birth, low birth weight, and fetal demise, are also more likely win women with hypertensive disorders.[9,10]

PATHOPHYSIOLOGY

The pathophysiology of hypertensive disorders in pregnancy is not understood fully. In pregnancy, the renin–angiotensin hormone system is upregulated and systemic vascular resistance decreases. As a result, blood pressure initially decreases starting as early as 7 weeks gestation. The decrease in diastolic blood pressure (DBP) tends to be greater than the decrease in systolic blood pressure (SBP). Maternal blood pressure begins to increase again in the third trimester.[11] The inciting event in the development of pregnancy-related hypertensive disorders is thought to be abnormal cytotrophoblast invasion of spiral arteries, leading to reduced uteroplacental perfusion. The resultant placental ischemia is assumed to cause an abnormal activation of the maternal vascular endothelium.[12]

The cardiovascular hemodynamics of hypertensive disorders are variable (**Table 1**).[13] In general, preeclampsia is associated with increased systemic vascular resistance, increased left ventricular afterload, and decreased cardiac output.[13,14] Conversely, based on a small cohort study using Doppler echocardiography in pregnancy, women with GHTN maintain low systemic vascular resistance and increased cardiac output.[14]

Preeclampsia involves a constellation of physiologic changes that include vasoconstriction, hemoconcentration, and possible ischemia in the placenta and other maternal organs. Vascular reactivity is owing to an imbalance and dysfunction in vasodilatory and vasoconstrictive substances. The resultant vasoconstriction decreases placental perfusion and perfusion of maternal organs, which can lead to end-organ damage. As renal blood flow decreases, so does the glomerular filtration rate. In rare cases, profoundly decreased renal perfusion can lead to acute tubular necrosis. Liver hematomas and rupture can occur in cases of preeclampsia, especially in conjunction with severe thrombocytopenia. The exact cause of eclamptic seizures is not well understood, but both hypertensive encephalopathy and ischemia secondary to vasoconstriction have been hypothesized. The visual changes (scotoma) often seen in women with preeclampsia may occur secondary to edema of the posterior cerebral hemispheres.[3]

Table 1		
Hemodynamic physiology of hypertensive disorders in pregnancy		
Disorder	**Systemic Vascular Resistance**	**Cardiac Output**
Pregnancy	Decreased	Increased
Gestational hypertension	Decreased	Increased
Preeclampsia	Increased	Decreased

PATIENT EVALUATION OVERVIEW
Diagnosis of Hypertensive Emergencies

Hypertension is defined as an SBP of greater than or equal to 140 mm Hg or DBP greater than or equal to 90 mm Hg on 2 occasions ($\geq$4 hours apart). Hypertension is considered severe with a SBP of 160 mm Hg or greater or a DBP of 110 mm Hg or greater.[1,11] As mentioned, preeclampsia is diagnosed in the presence of elevated blood pressure and either proteinuria ($\geq$300 mg of protein in a 24-h urine collection or protein to creatinine ratio of $\geq$0.3 mg/dL) or severe features as evidence of end-organ damage (**Box 1**). Severe forms of preeclampsia also include eclampsia and HELLP syndrome. HELLP is an acronym for hemolysis (H), elevated liver enzymes (EL) and low platelets (LP; see **Box 2**).[3]

Hypertension may be absent or mild in up to 50% of patients with HELLP syndrome. The differential diagnosis of HELLP includes acute fatty liver of pregnancy, gallbladder disease, lupus flare, and thrombotic thrombocytopenic purpura/hemolytic uremic syndrome. HELLP syndrome can be differentiated from these other conditions based on normal ammonia levels, mild renal insufficiency and anemia, and the presence of hypertension and proteinuria. A potential complication of HELLP syndrome is the development of a subcapsular liver hematoma. These patients often have phrenic nerve pain, and the diagnosis can be confirmed with imaging studies like computed tomography or abdominal ultrasonography.[3]

Hypertensive encephalopathy is a type of hypertensive emergency characterized by cerebral edema. This typically occurs in patients with SBP of greater than 220 mm Hg or DBP of greater than 120 mm Hg, although it can occur at lower blood pressures in pregnant women and those with newly increased blood pressures.[3,4] In hypertensive encephalopathy, there is a failure of the cerebral arteriolar constriction in response to increasing blood pressure. The signs and symptoms of hypertensive encephalopathy, including headache, confusion, and nausea, can develop over several days. Papilledema and retinal hemorrhages are frequently seen with fundoscopic examination in patients with hypertensive encephalopathy.[15] Signs of damage to other organs (eg, cardiac dysfunction or renal failure) may also be present.[3] Persistent evidence of neurologic deficits could indicate the presence of a stroke.[3]

PHARMACOLOGIC TREATMENT OPTIONS

The benefit of antihypertensive medication in mild-to-moderate CHTN remains uncertain and treatment is not recommended for persistent CHTN with a SBP of less than 160 mm Hg and a DBP of less than 105 mm Hg.[1,16] Likewise, antihypertensive medication is not

---

Box 2
Diagnosis of HELLP syndrome

- Evidence of hemolysis
  - Schistocytes on peripheral smear
  - Increased lactate dehydrogenase
  - Decreased haptoglobin
  - Increased total bilirubin ($\geq$1.2 mg/dL)
  - Decreased hematocrit (hemolysis) or increased hematocrit (hemoconcentration)
- Elevated aspartate and alanine aminotransferase ($\geq$70 IU/L)
- Thrombocytopenia (platelets <100,000/μL)

Abbreviation: HELLP, hemolysis, elevated liver enzymes, and low platelets.

recommended for GHTN or preeclampsia with a SBP of less than 160 mm Hg and a DBP of less than 110 mm Hg.[1] Treatment of mild to moderate hypertension results in a 50% decrease in the development of severe hypertension, but no difference in preeclampsia or other outcomes according to a Cochrane systematic review.[17] Conversely, treatment is recommended for severe hypertension (SBP $\geq$ 160 mm Hg and/or DBP >105–110 mm Hg) persisting for longer than 15 minutes.[18] All antihypertensive drugs cross the placenta and most are Food and Drug Administration category C (risks demonstrated in animal studies but no human studies have been performed; benefits may outweigh the risks). Changes to drug labeling, which include removal of the letter categories took effect June 30, 2015. The new labeling format will be used for all newly submitted drugs while changes to currently approved drugs will be phased in. The problems with medication use during pregnancy can be divided into teratogenicity (first trimester), fetotoxicity (throughout pregnancy), and breast feeding (**Table 2**).[19] Factors that modify the level of risk include agent, dose, and timing.[20] As is all too common, unplanned pregnancy often leads to delays in seeking prenatal care and either self-discontinuation or provider advice to stop taking prescription medications in the second trimester, at which point the risk of teratogenesis has already occurred.

Maternal hypertension during pregnancy has been associated with an increased risk of birth defects possibly owing to alterations in uterine blood flow.[21] These include congenital heart disease, esophageal atresia, and hypospadias.[21–23] In a systematic review and metaanalysis, Ramakrishnan and colleagues[21] found that congenital anomalies were more common in both treated and untreated hypertension, although the risk was greater in treated hypertension. Van Zutphen and colleagues[23] demonstrated a higher incidence of hypospadias in untreated hypertension and hypertension treated with nonselective β-blockers, specifically labetalol and propranolol. In this study, labetalol use may have been a surrogate for more severe hypertension. Alternatively, labetalol may affect the urethra during a critical period of development by altering uterine blood flow or may interfere with testosterone production by Leydig cells.

Few drugs have been sufficiently studied for use during pregnancy and there is a lack of randomized, placebo-controlled trials. Commonly recommended medications for the management of severe hypertension include intravenous labetalol and hydralazine, and oral nifedipine. Most guidelines recommend labetalol (66%) or hydralazine (33%) as first-line treatment and oral short-acting nifedipine as second-line treatment, although the ACOG now regards oral nifedipine as a first-line drug in the emergent treatment of severe hypertension.[18,24,25] Methyldopa, a centrally acting α2-adrenergic agonist, has also been suggested as a second-line agent for severe hypertensive crisis in some guidelines.[24] Methyldopa prevents vasoconstriction by replacing norepinephrine in the synaptic vesicles, thereby reducing catecholamine release and central sympathetic outflow. However, control is gradual over 6 to 8 hours, thus limiting its use in

Table 2		
Medication effects based on gestational age		
Gestational Age (From Last Menstrual Period), wk	**Effect**	**Consequence**
1–4	"All or nothing"	Either miscarriage or no effect.
5–12	Teratogenesis	Period of organ formation. Birth defects possible during this time.
12–42	Fetotoxicity	Organs completely formed. Possible damage to the brain and kidneys or impaired growth.

acute settings. More than 40 years of experience with methyldopa and follow-up in children up to 7.5 years old demonstrates the safety methyldopa during pregnancy, but multiple studies have demonstrated that other agents, namely labetalol, are more effective in controlling blood pressure. There are insufficient data to demonstrate the superiority of 1 drug over another; the choice of antihypertensive in the treatment of very high blood pressure during pregnancy depends on physician experience and knowledge of adverse effects. Drug characteristics and suggested dosing regimens are shown in **Tables 3** and **4** respectively.

In cases of refractory hypertension, labetalol infusion, nicardipine, and sodium nitroprusside are recommended. Refractory hypertension should be treated in conjunction with a specialist in maternal–fetal medicine or critical care. Nicardipine, like nifedipine, is a dihydropyridine calcium channel blocker. Nicardipine is indicated for use in severe hypertension. It has less negative ionotropic effect and is less likely to cause reflex tachycardia. Experience with nicardipine in pregnancy shows 91% success in decreasing blood pressure.[28] Sodium nitroprusside is a nonselective, direct nitric oxide donor available for use as an intravenous infusion because of its 3-minute duration of action. Sodium nitroprusside is used as a last resort, in part because of the risk of cyanide toxicity, which can occur after 24 to 48 hours. The risk of fetal cyanide poisoning is only theoretic.

Complete treatment of severely increased blood pressure should also include an assessment of fetal wellbeing and close monitoring of blood pressure, symptoms, and laboratory tests. Appropriate laboratory tests are hematocrit, platelet count, serum creatinine and transaminases. In addition, ultrasonography should be performed to assess fetal growth and amniotic fluid volume.[3]

TREATMENT COMPLICATIONS
Magnesium Toxicity

Magnesium is not an antihypertensive. It should be used for seizure prevention in preeclampsia with severe features and for neuroprotection when delivery is expected before 32 weeks gestation. The mechanism of action for magnesium sulfate in the prevention of seizures is unknown. It can be associated with several adverse effect and potential toxicities (**Table 5**).[3,29] Magnesium sulfate can cause uterine atony and increase the risk of postpartum hemorrhage.[3,29] Women receiving magnesium should be monitored closely and magnesium infusion stopped immediately if signs of toxicity develop. Magnesium toxicity can be treated with 10 mL of 10% calcium gluconate solution. Cardiopulmonary arrest, although rare, may require intubation and mechanical ventilation.[3]

Several case reports have documented adverse effects when combining magnesium and calcium channel blockers. One published case reported neuromuscular blockade,[30] and another case involved severe hypotension and subsequent maternal death.[1] However, a retrospective review of patients receiving both magnesium and nifedipine found no increase in neuromuscular weakness, neuromuscular blockade, or hypotension compared with controls.[31] Regardless, patients receiving both magnesium and nifedipine should be monitored closely given the potential for toxicities with the use of 2 calcium antagonists.[18]

Medications to Avoid in Pregnancy

There are several antihypertensive medications that are not recommended for use in pregnancy. Angiotensin-converting enzyme inhibitors, angiotensin receptor blockers, and mineralocorticoid receptor antagonists should be avoided without a specific

Table 3
Characteristics of antihypertensive drugs commonly used for severe hypertension during pregnancy

Drug (FDA Risk Category)	Mechanism	Perinatal Concerns	Side Effects
Labetalol (C)	Nonselective β-blocker and vascular α_1-receptor blocker	β-Blockers associated with congenital heart disease, cleft lip/palate, and open neural tube defects but causality not yet proven[26], generally regarded as safe Concern for growth restriction with atenolol but recent study suggests similar risk with labetalol[27] Fetal distress secondary to abrupt maternal hypotension Neonatal bradycardia and hypoglycemia	Caution in women with asthma (bronchoconstriction) Fatigue, lethargy, exercise intolerance, peripheral vasoconstriction, sleep disturbance
Hydralazine (C)	Direct vasodilator Relaxes arteriolar smooth muscle, exact mechanism unknown	Fetal distress secondary to abrupt maternal hypotension Cesarean section, abruption, APGAR <7 more common compared with other agents Rarely neonatal thrombocytopenia and neonatal lupus	Palpitations, tachycardia, headache, nausea/vomiting, flushing Side effects may mimic worsening preeclampsia Rarely polyneuropathy or drug-induced lupus
Nifedipine (C)	Dihydropyridine calcium channel blocker acting predominantly on the arterial smooth muscle	Increased liver clearance may require higher doses Fetal distress secondary to abrupt maternal hypotension	Tachycardia, palpitations, peripheral edema, headaches, flushing Risk of neuromuscular blockade, myocardial depression, and hypotension when combined with magnesium unsubstantiated Sublingual preparations associated with MI and death

Abbreviations: FDA, US Food and Drug Administration; MI, myocardial infarction.

Table 4
Initial approach to the management of severe hypertension

	Drug	
Labetalol	**Hydralazine**	**Nifedipine**
If BP remains ≥160 mm Hg systolic or ≥110 mm Hg diastolic for more than 15 min:		
Administer 20 mg IV over 2 min	Administer 5–10 mg IV over 2 min	Administer 10 mg orally
Repeat BP in:		
10 min	20 min	20 min
If BP remains ≥160 mm Hg systolic or ≥110 mm Hg diastolic:		
Administer 40 mg IV over 2 min	Administer 10 mg IV over 2 min	Administer 20 mg orally
Repeat BP in:		
10 min	20 min	20 min
If BP remains ≥160 mm Hg systolic or ≥110 mm Hg diastolic:		
Administer 80 mg IV over 2 min	Administer labetalol 20 mg IV over 2 min	Administer 20 mg orally
Repeat BP in:		
10 min	10 min	20 min
If BP remains ≥160 mm Hg systolic or ≥110 mm Hg diastolic:		
Administer hydralazine 10 mg IV over 2 min	Administer labetalol 40 mg IV over 2 min	Administer labetalol 40 mg IV over 2 min
Repeat BP in:		
20 min	10 min	10 min
If BP remains ≥160 mm Hg systolic or ≥110 mm Hg diastolic:		
Obtain emergency consultation and treat as recommended		

These algorithms are appropriate for antepartum, intrapartum, and postpartum severe hypertension.
Choice of agents should be guided by clinician experience and knowledge of adverse effect.
Management should also include physician notification, documentation, and fetal surveillance.
Once target BP is achieved, check BP every 10 minutes × 1 hour, then every 15 minutes × 1 hour, then every 30 minutes × 1 hour, then hourly for 4 hours.
Abbreviations: BP, blood pressure; IV, intravenous.
Adapted from American College of Obstetricians and Gynecologists. Committee opinion no. 623: emergent therapy for acute-onset, severe hypertension during pregnancy and the postpartum period. Obstet Gynecol 2015;125:521–5.

indication like proteinuric renal disease.[1] Angiotensin-converting enzyme inhibitors and angiotensin receptor blockers interfere with fetal renal hemodynamics leading to congenital anomalies in the first trimester and oligohydramnios, kidney damage, and death in the second and third trimesters. Mineralocorticoid receptor antagonists

Table 5
Magnesium toxicity associated with serum levels

Serum Magnesium Level (mg/dL)	Toxicity
8–12	Loss of deep tendon reflexes
10–12	Somnolence, Slurred speech
12–16	Respiratory paralysis
20–35	Cardiac arrest

like spironolactone can have anti-androgenic effects in pregnancy with feminization of the male fetus found in animal studies.[32] β-Blockers are commonly used antihypertensives in pregnancy, but there is ongoing debate about the risk of congenital anomalies and growth restriction (see **Table 3**).

EVALUATION OF OUTCOME
Goals of Treatment

The purpose of treatment of severe hypertension in pregnancy is to decrease maternal and fetal complications. Women with severely increased blood pressure are at risk of stroke, myocardial infarction, renal failure, uteroplacental insufficiency, placental abruption, and death.[11,33,34] Severe hypertension is the only modifiable end-organ complication of preeclampsia.[34] The blood pressure target for women with CHTN requiring antihypertensive therapy is to maintain a SBP of 160 mm Hg or less and a DBP of 105 mm Hg or less, or 160/110 mm Hg or less in GHTN and preeclampsia.[1] It is important to try to avoid an abrupt decrease in pressure which can lead to potential harmful fetal effects.[11] Therapy should aim to decrease mean arterial pressure by approximately 20% to 25% over minutes to hours then further decrease blood pressure to less than 160/110 mm Hg over the subsequent hours. The signs and symptoms of hypertensive encephalopathy (headache and confusion) often improve rapidly with treatment.

Fetal Evaluation

Monthly growth ultrasounds in the third trimester are recommended for women with CHTN. Umbilical artery Doppler velocimetry testing should be performed weekly if there is any evidence of fetal growth restriction or superimposed preeclampsia. In addition, antenatal fetal testing (e.g. nonstress testing) is suggested in women with CHTN and either coexisting need for medication, signs of fetal growth restriction, or superimposed preeclampsia.[1] Women with GHTN or preeclampsia in pregnancy should have ultrasounds to measure fetal growth, antenatal testing, twice weekly blood pressure checks, and weekly laboratory evaluations. Candidates for expectant management of preeclampsia with severe features require closer surveillance, including daily nonstress testing, weekly ultrasound for Doppler of the umbilical artery and amniotic fluid volume measurement, ultrasound every 2 to 3 weeks for growth, daily fetal movement counting, and periodic laboratory evaluation (frequency depends on patient stability).[3] Administration of corticosteroids for fetal lung maturity is recommended in women with preeclampsia at less than 34 weeks of gestation.[1]

Delivery Planning

Induction of labor is recommended for hypertensive disorders in pregnancy given the associated maternal and fetal morbidities in addition to the high risk of progression of disease. However, the optimal timing of delivery remains controversial. There have been no randomized, controlled trials to guide timing of delivery in women with CHTN. A cohort study of women with CHTN found that delivery at 38 to 39 weeks gestation was optimal for balancing fetal and neonatal risks.[35] The ACOG endorses delivery at 38 to 39 weeks for women with CHTN not requiring medication, 37 to 39 weeks for women controlled with medication, and 36 to 37 weeks for women with severe uncontrolled hypertension.[36]

A randomized, controlled trial in women with either GHTN or preeclampsia without severe features found that induction of labor at 37 weeks gestation was associated with a significant decrease in composite maternal morbidity as compared with expectant management.[37] The ACOG suggests delivery at 37 to 38 weeks for women with GHTN and induction of labor for preeclampsia without severe features at 37 weeks gestation.[36]

Both the ACOG and the Society for Maternal-Fetal Medicine recommend induction of labor at 34 weeks of gestation or greater in patients with preeclampsia with severe features.[36] A systematic review of induction of labor for preeclampsia with severe features before 34 weeks gestation found an association with decreased birth weight, greater rates of admission to the neonatal intensive care unit, longer neonatal hospitalization, and increased neonatal complications including intraventricular hemorrhage and respiratory distress syndrome.[38] However, induction of labor for preeclampsia with severe features is recommended before 34 weeks in women who are not candidates for expectant management (**Box 3**). In these women, delivery can be delayed for 48 hours for administration of corticosteroids for fetal lung maturity in the absence of uncontrollable severe hypertension, eclampsia, pulmonary edema, placental abruption, disseminated intravascular coagulation, or nonreassuring fetal status. The management of preeclampsia with severe features before viability (23–24 weeks in most centers) should involve consultation with a specialist in maternal–fetal medicine.

The mode of delivery should be decided based on the usual obstetric indications. Blood pressure should be controlled before delivery, especially in women undergoing cesarean section with general anesthesia because blood pressure can increase during endotracheal intubation. The use of neuraxial anesthesia is advised unless contraindicated by maternal thrombocytopenia.[1] The exact platelet level below which neuraxial anesthesia is contraindicated is controversial and varies from institution to institution based on platelet count (usually 50,000–100,000/μL), trend, and evidence of platelet dysfunction. Patients with severe thrombocytopenia (platelets <50,000) may require a platelet transfusion en route to the operating room if a cesarean delivery is indicated.[3]

Postpartum Management

Women with GHTN, preeclampsia, or CHTN with superimposed preeclampsia should have their blood pressure monitored for at least 72 hours postpartum and again 7 to

---

Box 3
Contraindications to expectant management of preeclampsia with severe features

- Severe hypertension refractory to medication
- Eclampsia
- Pulmonary edema
- Placental abruption
- Disseminated intravascular coagulation
- Thrombocytopenia (platelets <100,000/μL)
- Abnormal hepatic enzyme concentrations (twice normal)
- Renal dysfunction (creatinine >1.1 mg/dL or twice normal)
- Right upper quadrant or epigastric pain unresponsive to medication
- Unremitting cerebral or visual symptoms
- Nonreassuring fetal status
- Fetal demise

10 days after delivery.[1] Normalization of blood pressure typically occurs within 10 days of delivery in patients with pregnancy-related hypertension.[3] The ACOG recommends antihypertensive treatment in women with persistently increased blood pressures postpartum defined as SBP of 150 mm Hg or higher or DBP of 100 mm Hg or higher. Nonsteroidal antiinflammatory agents used to treat postpartum pain may exacerbate blood pressure owing to sodium and water retention.[39] An alternate analgesic can be considered in women with increased blood pressure that persists for more than 1 day postpartum.[1]

Women should be counseled and receive discharge instructions regarding the need to contact their health care provider if they develop warning signs or symptoms, including an unremitting headache, visual disturbances, or right upper quadrant pain. New-onset hypertensive disorders of pregnancy can also occur in the postpartum period. Postpartum women with newly elevated blood pressure should be evaluated and treated similarly to antenatal patients.[1]

Seizure prophylaxis is continued in patients with preeclampsia with severe features for 24 hours postpartum. Approximately 25% of cases of eclampsia occur in postpartum patients, and seizures can develop up to 4 weeks after delivery. Patients with preeclampsia with severe features are also at risk of developing pulmonary edema in the postpartum period. Furosemide can be used as deemed necessary in these patients.[3]

Women with pregnancies complicated by hypertensive disorders, especially preeclampsia requiring delivery at less than 34 weeks gestation, are at risk for the development of cardiovascular disease later in life. The ACOG suggests that women with a history of preeclampsia requiring a preterm delivery undergo yearly monitoring of blood pressure, lipids, fasting glucose, and body mass index.[1]

SUMMARY

Hypertensive disorders of pregnancy are associated with an increased risk of maternal and perinatal morbidity and mortality. Appropriate management of hypertension and its associated complications can optimize outcomes. Several antihypertensive agents can be used safely in pregnancy, although evidence from randomized controlled trials is lacking. A greater understanding of the pathophysiology, etiology, and natural history of hypertensive disorders in pregnancy would allow for improved prevention strategies and ultimate elimination of associated morbidity and mortality.

REFERENCES

1. American College of Obstetricians and Gynecologists, Task Force on Hypertension in Pregnancy. Hypertension in pregnancy. Report of the American College of Obstetricians and Gynecologists' task force on hypertension in pregnancy. Obstet Gynecol 2013;122(5):1122–31.
2. Duley L. Maternal mortality associated with hypertensive disorders of pregnancy in Africa, Asia, Latin America and the Caribbean. Br J Obstet Gynaecol 1992;99: 547–53.
3. Sibai BM. Hypertensive emergencies. In: Foley MR, Strong TH, Garite TJ, editors. Obstetric intensive care manual. 4th edition. New York: McGraw-Hill Education; 2014. p. 55–66.
4. Witlin AG, Friedman SA, Egerman RS, et al. Cerebrovascular disorders complicating pregnancy–beyond eclampsia. Am J Obstet Gynecol 1997;176:1139–48.
5. Creanga AA, Berg CJ, Syverson C, et al. Pregnancy-related mortality in the United States, 2006-2010. Obstet Gynecol 2015;125(1):5–12.

6. Kuklina EV, Ayala C, Callaghan WM. Hypertensive disorders and severe obstetric morbidity in the United States. Obstet Gynecol 2009;113(6):1299–306.
7. Wallis AB, Saftlas AF, Hsia J, et al. Secular trends in the rates of preeclampsia, eclampsia, and gestational hypertension, United States, 1987-2004. Am J Hypertens 2008;21:521–6.
8. Matthews TJ, Hamilton BE. Delayed childbearing: more women are having their first child later in life. NCHS Data Brief 2009;21:1–8.
9. Bramham K, Parnell B, Nelson-Piercy C, et al. Chronic hypertension and pregnancy outcomes: systematic review and meta-analysis. BMJ 2014;348:g2301.
10. Orbach H, Matok I, Gorodischer R, et al. Hypertension and antihypertensive drugs in pregnancy and perinatal outcomes. Am J Obstet Gynecol 2013; 208(4):e301–6.
11. Vidaeff AC, Carroll MA, Ramin SM. Acute hypertensive emergencies in pregnancy. Crit Care Med 2005;33(10):S307–12.
12. Granger JP, Alexander BT, Bennett WA, et al. Pathophysiology of pregnancy-induced hypertension. Am J Hypertens 2001;14(6 Pt 2):178S–85S.
13. Visser W, Wallenburg HC. Central hemodynamic observations in untreated preeclamptic patients. Hypertension 1991;17:1072–7.
14. Bosio PM, McKenna PJ, Conroy R, et al. Maternal central hemodynamics in hypertensive disorders of pregnancy. Obstet Gynecol 1999;94(6):978–84.
15. Sibai BM. On the brain in eclampsia. Hypertens Pregnancy 1994;13:111–2.
16. SMFM Publications Committee. SMFM statement: benefit of antihypertensive therapy for mild-to-moderate chronic hypertension during pregnancy remains uncertain. Am J Obstet Gynecol 2015;213(1):3–4.
17. Abalos E, Duley L, Steyn DW. Antihypertensive drug therapy for mild to moderate hypertension during pregnancy. Cochrane Database Syst Rev 2014;(2):CD002252.
18. American College of Obstetricians and Gynecologists. Committee opinion no. 623: emergent therapy for acute-onset, severe hypertension during pregnancy and the postpartum period. Obstet Gynecol 2015;125:521–5.
19. Redman CW. Hypertension in pregnancy: the NICE guidelines. Heart 2011; 97(23):1967–9.
20. Rakusan K. Drugs in pregnancy: implications for a cardiologist. Exp Clin Cardiol 2010;15(4):e100–3.
21. Ramakrishnan A, Lee LJ, Mitchell LE, et al. Maternal hypertension during pregnancy and the risk of congenital heart defects in offspring: a systematic review and meta-analysis. Pediatr Cardiol 2015;36(7):1442–51.
22. van Gelder M, Van Bennekom CM, Louik C, et al. Maternal hypertensive disorders, antihypertensive medication use, and the risk of birth defects: a case-control study. BJOG 2015;122(7):1002–9.
23. Van Zutphen AR, Werler MM, Browne MM, et al. Maternal hypertension, medication use, and hypospadias in the National Birth Defects Prevention Study. Obstet Gynecol 2014;123(2 Pt 1):309–17.
24. Al Khaja AJ, Sequeira RP, Al Khaja AK, et al. Drug treatment of hypertension in pregnancy: a critical review of adult guideline recommendations. J Hypertens 2014;32(3):454–63.
25. Duley I, Meher S, Jones L. Drugs for treatment of very high blood pressure during pregnancy. Cochrane Database Syst Rev 2013;(7):CD001449.
26. Meidahl Petersen K, Jimenez-Solem E, Andersen JT, et al. β-Blocker treatment during pregnancy and adverse pregnancy outcomes: a nationwide population-based cohort study. BMJ Open 2012;2(4):e001185.

27. Yakoob MY, Bateman BT, Ho E, et al. The risk of congenital malformations associated with β-blockers early in pregnancy: a meta-analysis. Hypertension 2013; 62(2):375–81.
28. Nij Bijvank SW, Duvekot JJ. Nicardipine for the treatment of severe hypertension in pregnancy: a review of the literature. Obstet Gynecol Surv 2010;65(5):341–7.
29. Lu JF, Nightingale CH. Magnesium sulfate in eclampsia and pre-eclampsia: pharmacokinetic principles. Clin Pharmacokinet 2000;38(4):305–14.
30. Ben-Ami M, Giladi Y, Shalev E. The combination of magnesium sulphate and nifedipine: a cause of neuromuscular blockade. Br J Obstet Gynaecol 1994; 101:262–3.
31. Magee LA, Miremadi S, Li J, et al. Therapy with both magnesium sulfate and nifedipine does not increase the risk of serious magnesium-related maternal side effects in women with preeclampsia. Am J Obstet Gynecol 2005;193(1): 153–63.
32. European Society of Gynecology (ESG), Association for European Paediatric Cardiology (AEPC), German Society for Gender Medicine (DGesGM). ESC guidelines on the management of cardiovascular diseases during pregnancy: the Task Force on the Management of Cardiovascular Diseases during Pregnancy of the European Society of Cardiology (ESC). Eur Heart J 2001;32(24):3147–97.
33. Martin JNJ, Thigpen BD, Moore RC, et al. Stroke and severe preeclampsia and eclampsia: a paradigm shift focusing on systolic blood pressure. Obstet Gynecol 2005;105:246–54.
34. Centre for Maternal and Child Enquiries (CMACE). Saving Mothers' Lives: reviewing maternal deaths to make motherhood safer: 2006–08. The eighth report on confidential enquiries into maternal deaths in the United Kingdom. BJOG 2011; 118:1–203.
35. Hutcheon JA, Lisonkova S, Magee LA, et al. Optimal timing of delivery in pregnancies with pre-existing hypertension. BJOG 2011;118(1):49–54.
36. American College of Obstetricians and Gynecologists. ACOG committee opinion no. 560: medically indicated late-preterm and early-term deliveries. Obstet Gynecol 2013;121(4):908–10.
37. Koopmans CM, Bijlenga D, Groen H, et al. Induction of labour versus expectant monitoring for gestational hypertension or mild pre-eclampsia after 36 weeks' gestation (HYPITAT): a multicentre, open-label randomised controlled trial. Lancet 2009;374(9694):979–88.
38. Churchill D, Duley L, Thornton JG, et al. Interventionist versus expectant care for severe pre-eclampsia between 24 and 34 weeks' gestation. Cochrane Database Syst Rev 2013;(7):CD003106.
39. Johnson AG, Nguyen TV, Day RO. Do nonsteroidal anti-inflammatory drugs affect blood pressure? A meta-analysis. Ann Intern Med 1994;121(4):289–300.

Neurologic Complications in Pregnancy

Mauricio Ruiz Cuero, MD[a], Panayiotis N. Varelas, MD, PhD[b],*

KEYWORDS

- Pregnancy • Stroke • Eclampsia • Status epilepticus • Brain death

KEY POINTS

- This article discusses the neurologic complications during pregnancy.
- This article analyzes and summarizes the most recent data about stroke, eclampsia, status epilepticus, neuromuscular disease, and brain death during pregnancy.
- This article emphasizes the physiopathology, epidemiology, and modality of treatments of the previously mentioned conditions.

INTRODUCTION

Obstetric practice occasionally mandates for admission of unstable patients to an intensive care unit. The reasons why such patients become critical can either be linked directly to the physiologic changes that occur during pregnancy and the puerperium or can be independent and coincidental. Because of its complexity and importance for the functional outcome of the mother, the nervous system, if affected, requires specialized management that in the past was offered by consulting services in neurology or neurosurgery. These days it may be better delivered by a team that includes neurointensivists and obstetricians in the neurosciences intensive care unit (NSU).

PREECLAMPSIA-ECLAMPSIA

Preeclampsia (PREC) is defined as the constellation of newly diagnosed hypertension (systolic/diastolic blood pressure [BP] ≥140/90 mm Hg on 2 occasions at least 4 hours apart after 20 weeks' gestation in a woman with previously normal BP; or BP ≥160/110 mm Hg, confirmed within a few minutes to facilitate timely antihypertensive

Disclosures: The authors have nothing to disclose.
[a] Neurocritical Care, Henry Ford Hospital, 2799 West Grand Boulevard, Detroit, MI 48202, USA;
[b] Neurosciences Critical Care Services, Neuro-Intensive Care Unit, Department of Neurology, Henry Ford Hospital, Wayne State University, K-11, 2799 West Grand Boulevard, Detroit, MI 48202, USA
* Corresponding author.
E-mail address: varelas@neuro.hfh.edu

Crit Care Clin 32 (2016) 43–59
http://dx.doi.org/10.1016/j.ccc.2015.08.002
0749-0704/16/$ – see front matter © 2016 Elsevier Inc. All rights reserved.

criticalcare.theclinics.com

treatment) and proteinuria (>300 mg/24 h or ≥1+ in dipstick testing; because of variability of qualitative determinations, this method is discouraged for diagnostic use unless other approaches are not readily available[1]; or protein/creatinine ratio ≥0.3). Alternatively, in the absence of proteinuria, it is defined by the presence of new onset of hypertension, as described earlier, with new onset of any of the following: serum creatinine level greater than 1.1 mg/dL or a doubling of the serum creatinine level in the absence of other renal disease, new onset of cerebral or visual symptoms, right upper quadrant or epigastric pain, pulmonary edema, thrombocytopenia less than,100,000/μL, or increased aspartate aminotransferase (AST) or alanine aminotransferase (ALT) level (to twice the normal concentration).[1] These systemic organ dysfunctions together with BP greater than or equal to 160/110 mm Hg should be considered severe features of PREC. Eclampsia (EC) is defined as seizures occurring before, during, or after delivery, and in up to 38% of cases it can occur without symptoms or signs of PREC.[1,2]

Epidemiology and Pathophysiology

In the developed world the incidence for PREC is 6% to 8% of pregnancies and for EC 1 in 2000 deliveries, although in the developing countries the numbers are much higher. EC confers a 1.8% maternal mortality and a 35% complication rate and in the United States ranks second only to embolic events as cause of maternal mortality.[3] PREC and its sequelae account for 20% to 50% of obstetric admissions to the NSU.[4]

The cause of PREC-EC is unknown. Pathophysiologic changes in the placental circulation, such as alteration of the ratio of prostacyclin/thromboxane/Flt-1, platelet activation/aggregation, and endothelial damage with fibrin deposition, lead to placental ischemia, diffuse maternal vasospasm, and microangiopathy.[5] The cerebral features include disruption of the capillary tight junctions and extravasation of fluids into the perivascular spaces, white matter edema, and cortical microhemorrhages or macrohemorrhages. Areas of infarction or ischemia are common, and are usually seen in the parieto-occipital watershed zones.[6,7] Because EC may develop at BPs that are considerably lower than those reported with hypertensive encephalopathy, a shift of the cerebral autoregulatory curve to the left or a reduced shift to the right, or loss of autoregulation with development of hydrostatic-vasogenic cerebral edema as a result of brain hyperperfusion at less than the necessary cerebral perfusion pressures, has been postulated.[8]

Clinical Presentation

Seizures are the hallmark of EC. They usually occur before childbirth or during labor, but in some women they occur as late as 10 to 23 days postpartum.[3] After the first 48 hours postpartum, clinicians should look for another cause, because only 3% of women experience late seizures from EC.[9] Seizures are usually generalized tonic-clonic, but occasionally may have a focal onset.[10] Headache, visual hallucinations, photophobia, confusion, and coma are other symptoms associated with EC.

Radiographic Features

In most EC cases computed tomography (CT) of the head is normal,[11] but in some it reveals focal lesions, such as cerebral edema, subarachnoid hemorrhage (SAH) or intraparenchymal hemorrhage, or, in patients with cortical blindness, occipital symmetric hypodensities.[6,12] MRI may show reversible low-signal intensities in T1 and high-signal intensities in T2-weighted images (with high apparent diffusion coefficient; ie, without diffusion restriction).[13]

Management

Management of patients with EC includes treatment of seizures and prevention of their recurrence, control of hypertension, timely delivery of the infant, and avoidance of further complications. Magnesium remains the cornerstone of treatment. One large international study of 10,141 pregnant women treated for PREC showed that Mg^{++} treatment conferred a 58% lower risk of EC, 33% lower risk for placental abruption, and a trend toward lower maternal mortality.[14] Superior Mg^{++} effectiveness in preventing and treating seizures in pregnant women has also been shown in 2 large randomized studies, comparing it with diazepam and phenytoin.[15,16] In addition, Mg^{++} was more effective than nimodipine for prophylaxis against seizures in women with severe PREC.[17]

Although several Mg^{++} treatment protocols exist, the one that is most commonly used in EC is a 4-g to 6-g intravenous (IV) bolus over 15 minutes, followed by 1 to 3 g/h IV infusion for at least 48 hours postpartum. If the treatment is used prophylactically in PREC, it can be stopped after 24 hours.[18] Careful monitoring for potential Mg^{++} toxicity should be done, preferably in an NSU setting. Loss of patellar reflexes, increasing drowsiness and dysarthria, muscle weakness, and respiratory depression, all should prompt for Mg^{++} level measurement, discontinuation of the infusion (therapeutic levels, 4–8 mEq/L) and use of calcium gluconate (1 g IV in 10% solution) in case of impending respiratory arrest. If seizures recur after Mg^{++} is given, either an extra 1 to 2g IV[16] or a loading dose of phenytoin (18 mg/kg IV at a maximum rate 50 mg/min) can be tried.

Blood pressure and volume control

The aim in BP control is not to normalize it but to bring it to a level of 140 to 150 mm Hg systolic and 90 to 100 mm Hg diastolic.[19] First-line therapies are IV hydralazine and labetalol, as well as oral nifedipine. Hydralazine has been successfully used in patients with PREC/EC as a 5-mg to 10-mg IV dose, which can be repeated every 20 minutes (as 10 mg, then 20 mg) and, if there is no appropriate response, followed by labetalol 40 mg IV in 10 minutes. If there is a response, the dose can be repeated every 6 hours. Labetalol can also be used, at a 20-mg IV dose, which can be repeated as a doubled dose (40 mg, then 80 mg) in 10-minute intervals and, if no appropriate response, followed by hydralazine 10 mg IV. Nifedipine can also be given as 10 mg by mouth and repeated as a 20 mg dose by mouth every 20 minutes, times 2 (if no appropriate response, then 40 mg IV labetalol is recommended). Specific order sets are provided in the most recent guidelines from the American College of Obstetricians and Gynecologists.[19] The dose of the antihypertensive medications is lowered after delivery and in most cases the drugs can be stopped within the first 6 weeks postpartum.[18] Ketanserin, a selective serotonin-2 receptor blocker, is considered inferior to hydralazine at reducing very high BP during pregnancy.[20] Angiotensin-converting enzyme inhibitors and angiotensin II receptor blockers should be avoided in PREC and EC.[21,22]

Volume status of patients with EC should be carefully assessed. Total fluid intake should not exceed 80 mL/h[22] and central venous pressure kept at less than 5 mm Hg,[18] because of a higher risk for pulmonary edema.

Intracranial dynamics

Cerebral edema and increased intracranial pressure management are not different from those for nonpregnant women. Adequate oxygenation, hyperventilation, mannitol infusion, loop diuretics, and correction of hyponatremia are general measures that can be taken, although their role in EC has not been tested in controlled studies.[11,23] Mannitol use during pregnancy should be judicious (US Food and Drug

Administration [FDA] category C medication). The same is true for loop diuretics, like furosemide. In serious or life-threatening situations during pregnancy, both drugs can be used.[24] We suggest that mannitol be used at 0.25 to 0.5 g/kg of prepregnancy maternal weight every 4 to 6 hours IV in such cases.

Termination of pregnancy

The time of delivery is decided by obstetricians. Patients should be hemodynamically stable and seizure free. The risk of prematurity should weigh against the risks for intrauterine growth restriction for the fetus and continuation of the eclamptic process for the mother. If the BP is controlled, pregnancy can be extended by an average of 2 weeks.[25] Maternal and fetal guidelines for expedited delivery or conservative management of severe PREC remote from term have been previously published.[1,26,27]

HEMOLYSIS, ELEVATED LIVER ENZYME LEVELS, AND LOW PLATELET LEVELS SYNDROME

The hemolysis, increased liver enzyme levels, and low platelet levels syndrome is a laboratory defined severe form of PREC. The acronym stands for hemolysis (anemia, increased bilirubin level, schistocytes in blood smear), increased liver enzyme levels (AST or ALT >70 U/L), and low platelet levels (<100,000/mm^3). It is associated with poor maternal (0%–24%) and perinatal (8%–60%) mortality caused by multisystem involvement. The incidence has been reported as 4% to 12% of patients with severe PREC, with higher risk in white, older patients.[28]

Pathophysiology and Clinical Features

Fibrin capillary deposition, organ hypoperfusion, microangiopathic hemolysis, and consumptive thrombocytopenia are the pathophysiologic mechanisms. Clinically, it presents as severe PREC with nausea, vomiting, and right upper quadrant pain. Hepatic hypoperfusion may lead to periportal and focal parenchymal necrosis, subcapsular hemorrhage, or hepatic rupture. Other complications include acute renal failure, adult respiratory distress syndrome, hypoglycemia, hyponatremia, diabetes insipidus, and organ hemorrhage (intracerebral, intraventricular, and retinal).[29–31] Ischemic cerebellar strokes have also been reported.[32,33] Cerebral angiography or transcranial Doppler may reveal diffuse vasospasm.[29]

Management

The treatment is similar to that of PREC, with prophylactic Mg^{++} sulfate infusion, antihypertensive therapy, and early delivery, as well as platelet and fresh frozen plasma (FFP) transfusions. Plasma exchange with FFP has been successfully used when thrombocytopenia, hemolysis, and organ dysfunction have persisted for greater than 72 hours postpartum.[34]

Dexamethasone leads to significantly shorter hospital length of stay, reduced mean interval to delivery, and greater mean birth weight. It was also significantly better than betamethasone for mean arterial pressure, platelet count, urinary output increase, and liver enzyme level increases.[35] Dexamethasone is administered as 10 mg IV every 6 hours for 2 doses, followed by 6 mg every 6 hours for another 2 doses. For more severe disease, the dose can be increased to 20 mg IV every 6 hours for 4 doses.[28]

MYASTHENIA GRAVIS

Myasthenia gravis (MG) is an autoimmune disorder of the neuromuscular junction, commonly affecting women in their third decade of life, who are of childbearing age.[36]

Clinical Course

The course of MG during pregnancy is at best unpredictable, with 10% to 19% of patients experiencing clinical worsening and most remaining stable or improving (59% and 22% respectively).[37,38] No correlation has been reported between the severity of MG before pregnancy and the risk for exacerbation during gestation. The highest risk for maternal mortality and clinical deterioration is within the first year after diagnosis, therefore women may consider delaying their pregnancies for at least 1 to 2 years after been diagnosed.[39] The first trimester and the puerperium are periods of MG exacerbation.[37,38]

MG may also affect the outcome of the fetus. Maternal antibodies crossing the placenta block the function of the fetal nicotinic acetylcholine receptor isoform, leading to arthrogryposis multiplex congenita, or more commonly to transient neonatal MG in 10% to 20% of infants.[40]

Management

The overall management of patients with MG should not change during pregnancy. However, vigilance is appropriate, because one or more complications occur during pregnancy in 21%, or during delivery in 41%, of patients.[38] Approximately 20% of patients develop respiratory crisis requiring mechanical ventilation caused by a combination of respiratory muscle weakness and decreased ability of the lungs to inflate fully secondary to the growing fetus. Acetylcholinesterase inhibitors, such as neostigmine 15 to 30 mg by mouth every 4 to 6 hours and pyridostigmine 30 to 60 mg by mouth 4 to 5 times daily remain the mainstay of treatment. Corticosteroids (prednisone, 40–80 mg by mouth daily) should be continued if they were started before conception.[41] There is only a slight increased risk for cleft lip and palate if taken during the first trimester and at high dose, and an increased risk of premature rupture of membranes and infectious complications.[36] Azathioprine, an FDA category D drug, is associated with teratogenicity in animals and, rarely, of malformations in humans.[37] A reasonable approach may be to delay the pregnancy until MG improvement permits reduction or discontinuation of this drug.[38] Methotrexate should be avoided during pregnancy because of a high risk for fetal abnormalities.[36] Thymectomy, performed before pregnancy, seems to correlate with a better course during subsequent pregnancy.[42] Plasmapheresis (PLA) and IV immunoglobulin (IVIG) are effective treatments in MG crisis[43–45] and can be used in pregnancy, either alone or sequentially.[37] PLA may carry a risk for premature labor because of large hormonal shifts and should be reserved for treatment of myasthenic crises.

Myasthenic crisis is usually caused by severe dysphagia and aspiration. It can be subtle and may be missed initially if arterial gases and pulmonary function tests are not done. Pao_2 (arterial partial pressure of O_2) less than 60 mm Hg and $Paco_2$ (arterial partial pressure of CO_2) 45 to 50 mm Hg, vital capacity less than 15 mL/kg, and negative inspiratory force less than -25 cm H_2O are indications for elective intubation and positive pressure ventilation. Tracheostomy is performed if the patient requires nasotracheal or orotracheal intubation for more than 2 weeks, but by that time greater than 50% of myasthenics are extubated.[46]

The striated muscles of the pelvic floor are involved and may fatigue during the expulsive efforts of the second stage of labor. Careful monitoring of the respiratory function during labor for signs of fatigue and hypoventilation, as well as parenteral administration of medications, is also recommended.[40] Outlet forceps or vacuum extraction should be used. In one study, cesarean sections were performed more frequently in women with MG.[47]

GUILLAIN-BARRÉ SYNDROME

Guillain-Barré syndrome (GBS), or acute inflammatory demyelinating polyradiculo-neuropathy (AIDP), is the most common cause of acute neuromuscular generalized paralysis. The diagnosis is made when there is progressive areflexic weakness (usually starting in the lower extremities), preceded in 50% of patients by back pain or leg paresthesias. Increased protein levels without cells in the cerebrospinal fluid (after the first week), prolonged distal latencies, and F-waves and antiganglioside antibodies strengthen the diagnosis.[48,49]

Epidemiology

The incidence of AIDP is approximately 0.75 to 2 in 100,000 per year and increases with age. Lower risk for GBS during pregnancy has been reported in a Swedish population (relative risk [RR], 0.86; 95% confidence interval [CI], 0.4–1.84).[50] However, nearly all of these cases occur in the second or third trimesters, but increased risk was also found during the 30 and 90 days postpartum (RR [95%CI], 2.21 [0.55–8.94] and 1.47 [0.54–3.99], respectively), suggesting a putative hormonal role.[50] Fetal survival is close to 96%, but premature delivery is common in severe GBS cases. Unlike MG, there is no GBS involvement of the fetus or neonate, except for 1 reported case.[51] In a review of 30 cases, 33% of patients required ventilatory support, but none died.[52]

Management

The management of GBS in pregnancy should be done in an NSU and is similar to that in nonpregnant patients. It is mainly supportive care until the patient regains her strength, with the addition of treatments that may change the natural course of the disease. These include PLA or IVIG, but pregnancy was an exclusion criterion for enrollment in the largest randomized studies.[53,54] Therefore, data during pregnancy are derived from case reports. GBS in pregnancy has been successfully treated with IVIG alone within 2 weeks from the onset of symptoms (0.4 g/kg/d for 5 days),[55–58] PLA alone (200–250 mL/kg over 4–6 sessions, up to a maximum of 402 mL/kg over 4 weeks),[59,60] or with a combination of IVIG-PLA (with PLA preceding).[51,61,62]

Close monitoring of the respiratory function with assessment of forced vital capacity (FVC) and the ability to cough and protect the airway is highly recommended in patients with GBS. The signs of respiratory failure are more insidious than in MG, because patients with autonomic dysfunction of the vagus nerve may lack the psychological feeling of breathlessness. If FVC is less than 1.5 L, the patient should be admitted to the NSU, and if less than 15 mL/kg, the patient should be intubated and mechanically ventilated. Another reason for NSU admission is dysautonomia. A temporary cardiac pacer is indicated in cases of bradyarrhythmia (usually after vagal stimulation following tracheal suction).

The risk of deep vein thrombosis and pulmonary embolism in patients with GBS has been estimated as between 2% and 13%.[63,64] The risk for venous thromboembolism among pregnant or postpartum women is 4.29 times higher than for nonpregnant women.[65–67] There is no reported estimate for when GBS and pregnancy coexist, but it may be inferred that it is even higher. Thus, pregnant patients with GBS should be treated for potential thromboembolic disease, although the optimal treatment and duration are unclear.

STROKE

Pregnancy is a physiologic state. However, it causes remodeling of the heart and all blood vessels. In animal studies, the walls of systemic arteries have shown a reduction in collagen and elastin content as well as a loss of distensibility. These biomechanical changes, along with the hemodynamic variation and changes in the levels of procoagulant factors, coagulation inhibitors, and other mediators of clot formation and lysis, make pregnancy a state of hypercoagulability. The incidence and the types of pregnancy-associated strokes remain open to question. The risk of stroke seems to be higher during the postpartum period. In the largest population-based study using the data of the Nationwide Inpatient Sample between 2006 and 2007, the rate of any stroke among antenatal hospitalizations was 0.22 per 1000 deliveries, 0.27 per 1000 deliveries for delivery hospitalizations, and 0.22 per 1000 deliveries among postpartum hospitalizations. The risk of stroke increased with age more than 35 years and was associated with African American race, migraine, thrombophilia or thrombocytopenia, systemic lupus erythematosus, heart disease, sickle cell disease, baseline or gestational hypertension, postpartum hemorrhage, PREC, transfusion, and postpartum infection.[68]

Specific pregnancy-related causes of stroke are presented in **Box 1**. The diagnostic work-up of stroke in pregnancy is similar to that in nonpregnant women, with the exception of radiological procedures and shielding for CT and angiography (first trimester, and especially the first month).[69,70]

Ischemic Stroke

Most of the strokes in pregnancy are attributed to arterial occlusions and cardioembolic events, which remain the most important cause.[71] Levels of procoagulant factors I, VII, VIII, IX, X, XII, and XIII increase during pregnancy, leading to a procoagulant state. In addition, the levels of some coagulation inhibitors, like antithrombin III or protein S, decrease during pregnancy, especially during the third trimester. Additional pregnancy-associated causes of stroke include peripartum cardiomyopathy, choriocarcinoma, and embolization of amniotic fluid or air. The incidence of ischemic stroke has been estimated at 3.5 per 100,000 per year[72] or 4.3 to 26 per 100,000 deliveries in the early 1990s.[71]

Although the frequency of the various causes of ischemic stroke is not known (see **Box 1**), it is widely thought that EC remains one of the commonest mechanisms, accounting for 24% to 47% of cases.[73,74] Within this spectrum should be included the posterior reversible encephalopathy syndrome (PRES) and the reversible cerebral vasoconstriction syndrome (RCVS), which often overlaps with PRES or EC and may also increase the risk for ischemic stroke and intracerebral hemorrhage (ICH).[75] Choriocarcinoma, a trophoblastic tumor associated with molar pregnancy, metastasizes in 20% of cases to the brain. The malignant cells invade the cerebral vessels, resulting either in local thrombosis and/or distal embolization or pseudoaneurysm formation and intracranial bleeding. Markedly increased serum beta–human chorionic gonadotrophin level is characteristic and measurement of this should be included in the diagnostic work-up of stroke during pregnancy.[76] Amniotic fluid embolism is a rare complication of labor in multiparous women, presenting with respiratory failure or cardiogenic shock and leading to disseminated intravascular coagulation (DIC). The neurologic symptoms consist mainly of encephalopathy or seizures in 10% to 20% of cases. Paradoxic cerebral embolism can also occur, the incidence of which is unknown. It can be diagnosed on cytologic examination of pulmonary artery catheter samples.[69,73] Other causes of cardioembolic stroke include peripartum cardiomyopathy, a rare dilating cardiomyopathy within the last month of pregnancy or 5 months postpartum, leading to stroke in 5% of cases. Anticoagulation is recommended. Another reason for anticoagulation is cervical artery dissection, reported in 6% to 7% of cases of pregnancy-related stroke. Antiphospholipid antibodies syndrome can lead to

---

Box 1
Causes of stroke during pregnancy

1. Ischemic
   Watershed
      Severe hypotension, Sheehan syndrome
   EC
   Choriocarcinoma
   Angiopathies
      Infectious: syphilis, borreliosis, tuberculosis, malaria, chlamydia pneumonia, herpes zoster, mycoses
      Inflammatory: collagen disorders, granulomatous angiitis of nervous system, sarcoidosis, Takayasu
      Noninflammatory: dissection, postpartum cerebral angiopathy, moyamoya, fibromuscular dysplasia, atherosclerosis, subarachnoid hemorrhage, vascular malformation
   Hematologic diseases
      Protein C, protein S, antithrombin III deficiency, factor V Leiden, homocystinuria, paraneoplastic coagulopathy, disseminated intravascular coagulation, thrombotic thrombocytopenic purpura, sickle cell disease, antiphospholipid antibodies, Sneddon syndrome
   Cardiac or pulmonary disorders
      Infective or marantic endocarditis, atrial myxoma, fibroelastoma, rheumatic heart disease, mitral valve prolapse, prosthetic valve, patent foramen ovale, amniotic fluid/fat/air embolism, atrial septal aneurysm, atrial fibrillation, acute myocardial infarct, dilated cardiomyopathy, peripartum cardiomyopathy, hereditary hemorrhagic telangiectasia
   Metabolic or channel dysfunction
      Cerebral Autosomal Dominant Arteriopathy with Subcortical infarcts and Leukoencephalopathy (CADASIL), migraine
   Air, fat, amniotic fluid embolism

2. Intracerebral hemorrhage
   EC, hypertension, cerebral venous and sinus thrombosis (discussed later), angiopathies (see earlier), choriocarcinoma, arteriovenous malformation (AVM), aneurysm, bacterial endocarditis, pituitary apoplexy, anticoagulation, cocaine abuse

3. Subarachnoid hemorrhage
   Aneurysm, AVM, EC, angiopathies (see earlier), choriocarcinoma, cerebral venous and sinus thrombosis (discussed later), bacterial endocarditis, pituitary apoplexy, anticoagulation, cocaine abuse

4. Cerebral venous and sinus thrombosis
   Hematologic diseases (see earlier), volume depletion, brain, sinus or mastoid infection, EC, cesarean section

Data from Refs.[24,69,124,125]

---

transient ischemic attacks or true infarcts, also occur during pregnancy or the puerperium, with or without the presence of a coexisting patent foramen ovale.[77] Low-dose heparin combined with aspirin in women with at least 2 fetal losses is recommended during pregnancy.[69]

The management of ischemic stroke during pregnancy requires admission to the NSU. Fibrinolysis has been considered a relative contraindication during pregnancy, but has been successfully used in 30 patients, 6 of whom received it intravenously and the rest intra-arterially. Complication rates and outcomes for children did not seem to be affected.[78,79] Use of aspirin during the first trimester is controversial.

However, low-dose aspirin (60–150 mg/d) during the second to third trimester was safely used in the CLASP (Collaborative Low dose Aspirin Study in Pregnancy) trial.[69,80]

Reported maternal mortality after ischemic stroke is 0% to 25% and one-third of patients have modified Rankin Disability Score less than 3. The risk for recurrence in subsequent pregnancies is estimated to be 2.3% within 5 years and is higher in patients with stroke of definite cause and during the postpartum period.[81]

Hemorrhagic Stroke

Hemorrhagic stroke is uncommon during pregnancy and the puerperium. The incidence from 3 population-based series is 0 to 6 per 100,000.[82] However, despite the low absolute risk, pregnancy increases the risk for hemorrhagic stroke much more than that for ischemic stroke. This risk increase is substantial during pregnancy (RR, 2.5) and peaks during the early postpartum period (RR, 28.5).[74] The major established causes of pregnancy-related cerebral hemorrhage are PREC/EC, followed by cerebral arteriovenous malformations (AVMs) and aneurysms.

The incidence of SAH during pregnancy is estimated at 20 per 100,000 deliveries and that of ICH at 4.6 to 6.1 per 100,000 deliveries. This incidence puts pregnant patients at higher risk for both compared with the nonpregnant population in the same age range.

The most common nontraumatic causes of SAH in pregnancy are AVMs and aneurysms in roughly equal proportions (see **Box 1**). The risk of aneurysmal rupture seems to increase several fold during pregnancy, increasing with gestational age until it peaks at 30 to 34 weeks. Dias and Sekhar[83] reported the mortality of pregnancy-associated aneurysmal SAH to be 35%, with a fetal mortality of 17%. In this retrospective study of 118 patients, 90% of aneurysmal bleeding occurred during pregnancy, 2% during labor, and 8% postpartum,[83] although others may not share this opinion.[84,85]

Causes of ICH during pregnancy included EC (44%), AVM, aneurysm, and cavernous angioma (12.5% each) or were undetermined (19%) in a large retrospective study[73] (see **Box 1**). In a US cohort, independent risk factors for pregnancy-related ICH included advanced maternal age, African American race, preexisting or gestational hypertension, PREC/EC, preexisting hypertension with superimposed PREC/EC, coagulopathy, and tobacco abuse.[86] AVMs are the most frequent cause of intracranial bleeding during pregnancy, constituting 4% to 5% of all ICH causes in nonpregnant women and up to 50% of ICHs in pregnant women.[87] Six percent of AVM-related ICH occurs during labor and 94% during pregnancy.[83,87]

The treatment of SAH or ICH is not different during pregnancy. Before and after securing the aneurysm, those patients should stay in the NSU. Clipping of the aneurysm can be achieved in any stage of pregnancy and is associated with lower maternal and fetal mortality.[69,83] Successful endovascular treatment with GDCs (Guglielmi Detachable Coils) has also been reported in a small number of patients,[88–90] but concerns have been raised regarding exposure to radiation and contrast (especially during the first trimester), systemic anticoagulation necessity, and partial obliteration of the aneurysm with subsequent need for follow-up angiographies.[84,89] Vasospasm can be treated with hypervolemia using crystalloids or colloids.[91] Triple H therapy (hypertension, hypervolemia, and hemodilution) has been abandoned in more recent guidelines for nonpregnant patients. Only hypertension is supported in those patients.[92] Pressors should be used with caution during pregnancy, because they diminish uteroplacental blood flow. Nimodipine has been used during pregnancy, but probably should be avoided because of teratogenic potential in animals.[91] There are no reported cases of balloon angioplasty for severe vasospasm after SAH, although it has been reported with EC-related vasospasm[93] and RCVS.[94] Delivery is preferred after the aneurysm is secured. Treatment at less than 24 weeks should be focused on the well-being of the mother. After 34 weeks, cesarean section followed by aneurysm exclusion may be preferred. Between 24 and 34 weeks, aneurysm exclusion with simultaneous fetal monitoring and, if needed, emergent cesarean section has been advocated. If, after treatment of the aneurysm, pregnancy continues to term, vaginal delivery is preferable.[91]

The treatment of AVMs does not differ from that in nonpregnant women.[69] In those patients with high operative risk or inoperable lesions, conservative management should be pursued during pregnancy, with stereotactic radiosurgery or embolization as options after delivery. Cesarean section is preferred in these cases. In low-risk, operable patients, surgery may improve the risks of poor outcome. The same can be said for surgery in comatose patients with large hematomas.[87]

Intraventricular hemorrhage can be treated with external ventricular drainage. Bilateral intraventricular thrombolysis with 5 mg/d of r-tPA (recombinant tissue Plasminogen Activator) in each side for 4 days has also been reported.[95]

SAH may result in 27% to 40% maternal mortality and may constitute the third most common cause of nonobstetric death in pregnancy.[69] The in-hospital mortality for pregnancy-related ICH is 20.3%[86] and the average maternal case-fatality rate can reach 30%.[96]

Cerebral Sinus Thrombosis

Cerebral venous thrombosis (CST) accounts for 6% to 64% of all pregnancy-associated strokes in large reported series.[82,96]

A high incidence of CST associated with pregnancy has been reported and is associated with a hypercoagulable state in 64% of cases and in 73% it occurred postpartum.[97] It presents with headache and ICH, with focal neurologic signs or seizures. CST occurs 1 to 4 weeks after childbirth and follows an otherwise normal delivery. Postdelivery headache should not be automatically attributed to spinal anesthesia during labor[98] and prompt diagnosis of CST should be made by MRI/magnetic resonance venography or CT venography.[99] Homocystine levels should be measured, because homocystinemia may be associated with peripartum CST.[100] A more extensive hypercoagulability work-up is also optional (see **Box 1**).

IV heparin, fluid administration, antibiotics for infection, and measures to reduce the increased intracranial pressure are all used in CST. Oral anticoagulation is usually given for 6 months in those patients with idiopathic venous thrombosis and indefinitely in those with a persistent or familial thrombophilic state. The risk for hemorrhagic conversion has been used as the major argument against anticoagulation and the only data from randomized studies are in nonpregnant populations.[101,102] In an uncontrolled study, 24% of patients with CST complicating pregnancy who received heparin died, compared with 45% of untreated patients. One fatal hemorrhage occurred in the group with heparin.[103] Combined intrathrombus r-tPA and IV heparin with good outcomes has also been reported.[104,105]

Mortality from pregnancy-associate CST is 10% to 50%,[99] with case-fatality rate in the range of 4% to 36%.[106]

STATUS EPILEPTICUS

Most epileptic women have unchanged seizure frequency during pregnancy. Exacerbation of seizures can occur in 37% of pregnant epileptics.[107] Status epilepticus (SE) during pregnancy is rare. In a 1999 review of the English literature, 19 case reports were identified. SE was previously experienced in only 3 of 19 women and occurred in the third trimester in 74% of cases.[108] In a large prospective antiepileptic drugs and pregnancy registry (EURAP [European Registry of Antiepileptic Drugs and Pregnancy]), 36 of 1956 pregnancies developed SE (12 of them convulsive; 1.8%). Thirteen occurred in the first, 11 in the second, and 13 in the third trimester (1 during delivery). SE resulted in 1 stillbirth and no miscarriages or maternal deaths.[109]

If a nonepileptic pregnant woman develops new-onset seizures, EC should be excluded in the third trimester and similar causes of seizures (tumor, stroke, central nervous system infection, trauma, hypoglycemia), as in nonpregnant women, should be sought.[110] The most common cause is thought to be drug noncompliance (caused by fear for teratogenicity) and changes in drug level. However, in the EURAP study, no particular risk factor for SE was identified and antiepileptic drugs were either unchanged since conception or the numbers or dosages were increased in 35 of 36 cases before developing SE.[109] Increased plasma clearance of antiepileptic drugs with advancing gestation has to be balanced against an increased ratio of unbound free to total drug levels.[111–113] Although acidosis and hypoxia from SE may double maternal mortality, increase the risk for spontaneous abortion by 50%, and lead to fetal or neonatal death in 48% of cases,[112,114] more recent data showed that only 1 of 36 pregnancies complicated by SE ended with stillbirth and none was associated with maternal mortality.[109]

The SE treatment algorithm does not differ from that in nonpregnant women[115,116] and its goal is to stop the electrical and clinical seizure activity as soon as possible and support the mother and fetus.[117,118] Administration of IV antiepileptic drugs should not be delayed, even during the embryogenesis period. Medications that are highly protein bound should initially be administered in lower dose to avoid toxic free drug levels.[119] Reduced loading doses of phenytoin are used (10–15 mg/kg), but eventually full dosages can be given if seizures continue.[115,116] Delivery should be started only for obstetric reasons. The neonate should be supported in the neonatal intensive care unit if benzodiazepines or barbiturates are given.

BRAIN DEATH

The criteria of diagnosing brain death during pregnancy do not differ from those for nonpregnant women. However, there are several controversial ethical issues for supporting the mother until or beyond the fetus is viable (24 weeks). Her right for autonomy should be balanced against fetal rights for survival. Her wishes and, if never expressed, those of the next of kin, and particularly those of the biological father of the fetus, should be respected.[120]

How often this catastrophic event happens is unknown. In a recent review, 30 cases were reported between 1982 and 2010. The mean gestational age at the time of brain death and the mean gestational age at delivery were 22 and 29.5 weeks, respectively. Twelve viable infants were born and survived the neonatal period.[121] Bernstein and colleagues[122] reported the case with the longest duration of post–brain death support, which is also the one with the earliest gestational age when brain death occurred (15 weeks' gestation). She was supported for 107 days, when, because of fetal distress, she delivered a 1550-g infant.

The myriad problems that should be addressed include continuous hemodynamic support and monitoring; use of pressors (dobutamine, dopamine, or norepinephrine) and IV fluids; left lateral recumbent position placement; monitoring of volume status with Swan-Ganz catheterization; continuous ventilatory support, with a $Paco_2$ goal of 30 to 35 mm Hg; enteral or parenteral nutrition; tocolytic treatment, preferentially with Mg^{++}; physiologic vasopressin infusion rates for diabetes insipidus; hydrocortisone and thyroxine replacement for panhypopituitarism; glucose monitoring and insulin-need adjustments; treatment of infections; and rewarming of the frequently poikilo-thermic mother. In addition, continuous fetal monitoring and psychological support of the family and the medical and nursing staff involved in the care of a dead patient used, in effect, as a fetal container[120] or incubator[123] is often needed during the pro-longed NSU course.

REFERENCES

1. American College of Obstetricians and Gynecologists, Task Force on Hyperten-sion in Pregnancy. Report of the American College of Obstetricians and Gyne-cologists' Task Force on Hypertension in Pregnancy. Obstet Gynecol 2013;122: 1122–31.
2. Mushambi MC, Halligan AW, Williamson K. Recent developments in the patho-physiology and management of pre-eclampsia. Br J Anaesth 1996;76:133–48.
3. Douglas KA, Redman CW. Eclampsia in the United Kingdom. BMJ 1994;309: 1395–400.
4. Mabie WC, Sibai BM. Treatment in an obstetric intensive care unit. Am J Obstet Gynecol 1990;162:1–4.
5. Levine RJ, Karumanchi SA. Circulating angiogenic factors in preeclampsia. Clin Obstet Gynecol 2005;48:372–86.
6. Ramin KD. The prevention and management of eclampsia. Obstet Gynecol Clin North Am 1999;26:489–503, ix.
7. Kaplan PW. Neurologic issues in eclampsia. Rev Neurol (Paris) 1999;155: 335–41.
8. Cipolla MJ. Cerebrovascular function in pregnancy and eclampsia. Hypertension 2007;50:14–24.
9. Miles JF Jr, Martin JN Jr, Blake PG, et al. Postpartum eclampsia: a recurring perinatal dilemma. Obstet Gynecol 1990;76:328–31.
10. Porapakkham S. An epidemiologic study of eclampsia. Obstet Gynecol 1979; 54:26–30.
11. Thomas SV. Neurological aspects of eclampsia. J Neurol Sci 1998;155:37–43.
12. Sibai BM. Eclampsia. VI. Maternal-perinatal outcome in 254 consecutive cases. Am J Obstet Gynecol 1990;163:1049–54 [discussion: 1054–5].
13. Zak IT, Dulai HS, Kish KK. Imaging of neurologic disorders associated with pregnancy and the postpartum period. Radiographics 2007;27:95–108.
14. Altman D, Carroli G, Duley L, et al. Do women with pre-eclampsia, and their babies, benefit from magnesium sulphate? The Magpie Trial: a randomised placebo-controlled trial. Lancet 2002;359:1877–90.
15. Which anticonvulsant for women with eclampsia? Evidence from the Collabora-tive Eclampsia Trial. Lancet 1995;345:1455–63.
16. Lucas MJ, Leveno KJ, Cunningham FG. A comparison of magnesium sulfate with phenytoin for the prevention of eclampsia. N Engl J Med 1995;333:201–5.
17. Belfort MA, Anthony J, Saade GR, et al. A comparison of magnesium sulfate and nimodipine for the prevention of eclampsia. N Engl J Med 2003;348:304–11.
18. Walker JJ. Pre-eclampsia. Lancet 2000;356:1260–5.
19. Committee on Obstetric Practice. Committee opinion no. 623: emergent therapy for acute-onset, severe hypertension during pregnancy and the postpartum period. Obstet Gynecol 2015;125:521–5.
20. Duley L, Henderson-Smart DJ. Drugs for rapid treatment of very high blood pressure during pregnancy. Cochrane Database Syst Rev 2000;(2):CD001449.

21. Bouba I, Makrydimas G, Kalaitzidis R, et al. Interaction between the polymorphisms of the renin-angiotensin system in preeclampsia. Eur J Obstet Gynecol Reprod Biol 2003;110:8–11.

22. von Dadelszen P, Menzies J, Gilgoff S, et al. Evidence-based management for preeclampsia. Front Biosci 2007;12:2876–89.

23. Lapinsky SE, Kruczynski K, Slutsky AS. Critical care in the pregnant patient. Am J Respir Crit Care Med 1995;152:427–55.

24. Donaldson JO. Neurologic emergencies in pregnancy. Obstet Gynecol Clin North Am 1991;18:199–212.

25. Magee LA, Ornstein MP, von Dadelszen P. Fortnightly review: management of hypertension in pregnancy. BMJ 1999;318:1332–6.

26. Repke JT, Robinson JN. The prevention and management of pre-eclampsia and eclampsia. Int J Gynaecol Obstet 1998;62:1–9.

27. Gillon TE, Pels A, von Dadelszen P, et al. Hypertensive disorders of pregnancy: a systematic review of international clinical practice guidelines. PLoS One 2014; 9:e113715.

28. O'Brien JM, Barton JR. Controversies with the diagnosis and management of HELLP syndrome. Clin Obstet Gynecol 2005;48:460–77.

29. Knopp U, Kehler U, Rickmann H, et al. Cerebral haemodynamic pathologies in HELLP syndrome. Clin Neurol Neurosurg 2003;105:256–61.

30. Murphy MA, Ayazifar M. Permanent visual deficits secondary to the HELLP syndrome. J Neuroophthalmol 2005;25:122–7.

31. Hirashima C, Ohkuchi A, Matsubara S, et al. Hydrocephalus after intraventricular hemorrhage in eclamptic woman with HELLP syndrome. Hypertens Pregnancy 2006;25:255–7.

32. Soh Y, Yasuhi I, Nakayama D, et al. A case of postpartum cerebellar infarction with hemolysis, elevated liver enzymes, low platelets (HELLP) syndrome. Gynecol Obstet Invest 2002;53:240–2.

33. Altamura C, Vasapollo B, Tibuzzi F, et al. Postpartum cerebellar infarction and haemolysis, elevated liver enzymes, low platelet (HELLP) syndrome. Neurol Sci 2005;26:40–2.

34. Martin JN Jr, Perry KG Jr, Roberts WE, et al. Plasma exchange for preeclampsia: III. Immediate peripartal utilization for selected patients with HELLP syndrome. J Clin Apher 1994;9:162–5.

35. Matchaba P, Moodley J. Corticosteroids for HELLP syndrome in pregnancy. Cochrane Database Syst Rev 2004;(1):CD002076.

36. Ferrero S, Pretta S, Nicoletti A, et al. Myasthenia gravis: management issues during pregnancy. Eur J Obstet Gynecol Reprod Biol 2005;121:129–38.

37. Batocchi AP, Majolini L, Evoli A, et al. Course and treatment of myasthenia gravis during pregnancy. Neurology 1999;52:447–52.

38. Hoff JM, Daltveit AK, Gilhus NE. Myasthenia gravis in pregnancy and birth: identifying risk factors, optimising care. Eur J Neurol 2007;14:38–43.

39. Djelmis J, Sostarko M, Mayer D, et al. Myasthenia gravis in pregnancy: report on 69 cases. Eur J Obstet Gynecol Reprod Biol 2002;104:21–5.

40. Stafford IP, Dildy GA. Myasthenia gravis and pregnancy. Clin Obstet Gynecol 2005;48:48–56.

41. Daskalakis GJ, Papageorgiou IS, Petrogiannis ND, et al. Myasthenia gravis and pregnancy. Eur J Obstet Gynecol Reprod Biol 2000;89:201–4.

42. Roth TC, Raths J, Carboni G, et al. Effect of pregnancy and birth on the course of myasthenia gravis before or after transsternal radical thymectomy. Eur J Cardiothorac Surg 2006;29:231–5.

43. Qureshi AI, Choudhry MA, Akbar MS, et al. Plasma exchange versus intravenous immunoglobulin treatment in myasthenic crisis. Neurology 1999;52:629–32.

44. Achiron A, Barak Y, Miron S, et al. Immunoglobulin treatment in refractory myasthenia gravis. Muscle Nerve 2000;23:551–5.

45. Carr SR, Gilchrist JM, Abuelo DN, et al. Treatment of antenatal myasthenia gravis. Obstet Gynecol 1991;78:485–9.

46. Thomas CE, Mayer SA, Gungor Y, et al. Myasthenic crisis: clinical features, mortality, complications, and risk factors for prolonged intubation. Neurology 1997; 48:1253–60.

47. Hoff JM, Daltveit AK, Gilhus NE. Myasthenia gravis: consequences for pregnancy, delivery, and the newborn. Neurology 2003;61:1362–6.

48. Ho T, Griffin J. Guillain-Barre syndrome. Curr Opin Neurol 1999;12:389–94.

49. Ropper AH. The Guillain-Barre syndrome. N Engl J Med 1992;326:1130–6.

50. Jiang GX, de Pedro-Cuesta J, Strigard K, et al. Pregnancy and Guillain-Barre syndrome: a nationwide register cohort study. Neuroepidemiology 1996;15: 192–200.

51. Luijckx GJ, Vles J, de Baets M, et al. Guillain-Barre syndrome in mother and newborn child. Lancet 1997;349:27.

52. Chan LY, Tsui MH, Leung TN. Guillain-Barre syndrome in pregnancy. Acta Obstet Gynecol Scand 2004;83:319–25.

53. van der Meche FG, Schmitz PI. A randomized trial comparing intravenous immune globulin and plasma exchange in Guillain-Barre syndrome. Dutch Guillain-Barre Study Group. N Engl J Med 1992;326:1123–9.

54. Randomised trial of plasma exchange, intravenous immunoglobulin, and combined treatments in Guillain-Barre syndrome. Plasma Exchange/Sandoglobulin Guillain-Barre Syndrome Trial Group. Lancet 1997;349:225–30.

55. Yamada H, Noro N, Kato EH, et al. Massive intravenous immunoglobulin treatment in pregnancy complicated by Guillain-Barre Syndrome. Eur J Obstet Gynecol Reprod Biol 2001;97:101–4.

56. Kocabas S, Karaman S, Firat V, et al. Anesthetic management of Guillain-Barre syndrome in pregnancy. J Clin Anesth 2007;19:299–302.

57. Vijayaraghavan J, Vasudevan D, Sadique N, et al. A rare case of Guillain-Barre syndrome with pregnancy. J Indian Med Assoc 2006;104:269–70.

58. Vaduva C, de Seze J, Volatron AC, et al. Severe Guillain-Barre syndrome and pregnancy: two cases with rapid improvement post-partum. Rev Neurol (Paris) 2006;162:358–62 [in French].

59. Gautier PE, Hantson P, Vekemans MC, et al. Intensive care management of Guillain-Barre syndrome during pregnancy. Intensive Care Med 1990;16:460–2.

60. Goyal V, Misra BK, Singh S, et al. Acute inflammatory demyelinating polyneuropathy in patients with pregnancy. Neurol India 2004;52:283–4.

61. Yaginuma Y, Kawamura M, Ishikawa M. Landry-Guillain-Barre-Strohl syndrome in pregnancy. J Obstet Gynaecol Res 1996;22:47–9.

62. Brooks H, Christian AS, May AE. Pregnancy, anaesthesia and Guillain Barre syndrome. Anaesthesia 2000;55:894–8.

63. Ferner R, Barnett M, Hughes RA. Management of Guillain-Barre syndrome. Br J Hosp Med 1987;38:525–8, 530.

64. Ropper AH. Critical care of Guillain-Barre syndrome. In: Ropper AH, editor. Neurological and neurosurgical intensive care. 3rd edition. New York: Raven Press; 1993. p. 363–82.

65. Demers C, Ginsberg JS. Deep venous thrombosis and pulmonary embolism in pregnancy. Clin Chest Med 1992;13:645–56.

66. Barbour LA. Current concepts of anticoagulant therapy in pregnancy. Obstet Gynecol Clin North Am 1997;24:499–521.
67. Heit JA, Kobbervig CE, James AH, et al. Trends in the incidence of venous thromboembolism during pregnancy or postpartum: a 30-year population-based study. Ann Intern Med 2005;143:697–706.
68. James AH, Bushnell CD, Jamison MG, et al. Incidence and risk factors for stroke in pregnancy and the puerperium. Obstet Gynecol 2005;106:509–16.
69. Mas JL, Lamy C. Stroke in pregnancy and the puerperium. J Neurol 1998;245:305–13.
70. Feske SK. Stroke in pregnancy. Semin Neurol 2007;27:442–52.
71. Jaigobin C, Silver FL. Stroke and pregnancy. Stroke 2000;31:2948–51.
72. Wiebers DO, Whisnant JP. The incidence of stroke among pregnant women in Rochester, Minn, 1955 through 1979. JAMA 1985;254:3055–7.
73. Sharshar T, Lamy C, Mas JL. Incidence and causes of strokes associated with pregnancy and puerperium. A study in public hospitals of Ile de France. Stroke in Pregnancy Study Group. Stroke 1995;26:930–6.
74. Kittner SJ, Stern BJ, Feeser BR, et al. Pregnancy and the risk of stroke. N Engl J Med 1996;335:768–74.
75. Skeik N, Porten BR, Kadkhodayan Y, et al. Postpartum reversible cerebral vaso-constriction syndrome: review and analysis of the current data. Vasc Med 2015;20:256–65.
76. Saad N, Tang YM, Sclavos E, et al. Metastatic choriocarcinoma: a rare cause of stroke in the young adult. Australas Radiol 2006;50:481–3.
77. Giberti L, Bino G, Tanganelli P. Pregnancy, patent foramen ovale and stroke: a case of pseudoperipheral facial palsy. Neurol Sci 2005;26:43–5.
78. De Keyser J, Gdovinova Z, Uyttenboogaart M, et al. Intravenous alteplase for stroke: beyond the guidelines and in particular clinical situations. Stroke 2007;38:2612–8.
79. Selim MH, Molina CA. The use of tissue plasminogen-activator in pregnancy: a taboo treatment or a time to think out of the box. Stroke 2013;44:868–9.
80. CLASP: a randomised trial of low-dose aspirin for the prevention and treatment of pre-eclampsia among 9364 pregnant women. CLASP (Collaborative Low-dose Aspirin Study in Pregnancy) Collaborative Group. Lancet 1994;343:619–29.
81. Lamy C, Hamon JB, Coste J, et al. Ischemic stroke in young women: risk of recurrence during subsequent pregnancies. French Study Group on Stroke in Pregnancy. Neurology 2000;55:269–74.
82. Feske SK, Singhal AB. Cerebrovascular disorders complicating pregnancy. Continuum 2014;20:80–99.
83. Dias MS, Sekhar LN. Intracranial hemorrhage from aneurysms and arteriove-nous malformations during pregnancy and the puerperium. Neurosurgery 1990;27:855–65 [discussion: 865–6].
84. Marshman LA, Aspoas AR, Rai MS, et al. The implications of ISAT and ISUIA for the management of cerebral aneurysms during pregnancy. Neurosurg Rev 2007;30:177–80 [discussion: 180].
85. Stoodley MA, Macdonald RL, Weir BK. Pregnancy and intracranial aneurysms. Neurosurg Clin North Am 1998;9:549–56.
86. Bateman BT, Schumacher HC, Bushnell CD, et al. Intracerebral hemorrhage in pregnancy: frequency, risk factors, and outcome. Neurology 2006;67:424–9.
87. Trivedi RA, Kirkpatrick PJ. Arteriovenous malformations of the cerebral circula-tion that rupture in pregnancy. J Obstet Gynaecol 2003;23:484–9.

88. Meyers PM, Halbach VV, Malek AM, et al. Endovascular treatment of cerebral artery aneurysms during pregnancy: report of three cases. AJNR Am J Neuroradiol 2000;21:1306–11.

89. Kizilkilic O, Albayram S, Adaletli I, et al. Endovascular treatment of ruptured intracranial aneurysms during pregnancy: report of three cases. Arch Gynecol Obstet 2003;268:325–8.

90. Piotin M, de Souza Filho CB, Kothimbakam R, et al. Endovascular treatment of acutely ruptured intracranial aneurysms in pregnancy. Am J Obstet Gynecol 2001;185:1261–2.

91. Selo-Ojeme DO, Marshman LA, Ikomi A, et al. Aneurysmal subarachnoid haemorrhage in pregnancy. Eur J Obstet Gynecol Reprod Biol 2004;116:131–43.

92. Diringer MN, Bleck TP, Claude Hemphill J 3rd, et al. Critical care management of patients following aneurysmal subarachnoid hemorrhage: recommendations from the Neurocritical Care Society's Multidisciplinary Consensus Conference. Neurocrit Care 2011;15:211–40.

93. Ringer AJ, Qureshi AI, Kim SH, et al. Angioplasty for cerebral vasospasm from eclampsia. Surg Neurol 2001;56:373–8 [discussion: 378–9].

94. Fugate JE, Wijdicks EF, Parisi JE, et al. Fulminant postpartum cerebral vasoconstriction syndrome. Arch Neurol 2012;69:111–7.

95. Newman P, Al-Memar A. Intraventricular haemorrhage in pregnancy due to moya-moya disease. J Neurol Neurosurg Psychiatry 1998;64:686.

96. Liang CC, Chang SD, Lai SL, et al. Stroke complicating pregnancy and the puerperium. Eur J Neurol 2006;13:1256–60.

97. Jeng JS, Tang SC, Yip PK. Stroke in women of reproductive age: comparison between stroke related and unrelated to pregnancy. J Neurol Sci 2004;221:25–9.

98. Kapessidou Y, Vokaer M, Laureys M, et al. Case report: cerebral vein thrombosis after subarachnoid analgesia for labour. Can J Anaesth 2006;53:1015–9.

99. Bousser MG. Cerebral venous thrombosis: nothing, heparin, or local thrombolysis? Stroke 1999;30:481–3.

100. Vignazia GL, La Mura F, Gaidano G, et al. Post gravidic superior sagittal sinus thrombosis with elevated levels of homocystinemia. Minerva Anestesiol 2004;70:831–6.

101. Einhaupl KM, Villringer A, Meister W, et al. Heparin treatment in sinus venous thrombosis. Lancet 1991;338:597–600.

102. de Bruijn SF, Stam J. Randomized, placebo-controlled trial of anticoagulant treatment with low-molecular-weight heparin for cerebral sinus thrombosis. Stroke 1999;30:484–8.

103. Srinivasan K. Puerperal cerebral venous and arterial thrombosis. Semin Neurol 1988;8:222–5.

104. Frey JL, Muro GJ, McDougall CG, et al. Cerebral venous thrombosis: combined intrathrombus rtPA and intravenous heparin. Stroke 1999;30:489–94.

105. Weatherby SJ, Edwards NC, West R, et al. Good outcome in early pregnancy following direct thrombolysis for cerebral venous sinus thrombosis. J Neurol 2003;250:1372–3.

106. Canhao P, Ferro JM, Lindgren AG, et al. Causes and predictors of death in cerebral venous thrombosis. Stroke 2005;36:1720–5.

107. Schmidt D, Canger R, Avanzini G, et al. Change of seizure frequency in pregnant epileptic women. J Neurol Neurosurg Psychiatry 1983;46:751–5.

108. Licht EA, Sankar R. Status epilepticus during pregnancy. A case report. J Reprod Med 1999;44:370–2.

109. Seizure control and treatment in pregnancy: observations from the EURAP epilepsy pregnancy registry. Neurology 2006;66:354–60.
110. Michalsen A, Henze T, Wagner D, et al. Status epilepticus late in pregnancy–eclampsia or subarachnoid hemorrhage? Anasthesiol Intensivmed Notfallmed Schmerzther 1997;32:380–4 [in German].
111. Morrell MJ. The new antiepileptic drugs and women: efficacy, reproductive health, pregnancy, and fetal outcome. Epilepsia 1996;37:S34–44.
112. Donaldson J. Neurologic complications. In: Burrow G, Duffy T, editors. Medical complications during pregnancy. 5th edition. Philadelphia: WB Saunders; 1999. p. 401–14.
113. Yerby MS, Friel PN, McCormick K. Antiepileptic drug disposition during pregnancy. Neurology 1992;42:12–6.
114. Teramo K, Hiilesmaa V. Pregnancy and fetal complications in epileptic pregnancies: review of the literature. In: Janz D, editor. Epilepsy, pregnancy and the child. New York: Raven Press; 1982. p. 53–9.
115. Varelas PN, Mirski MA. Seizures in the adult intensive care unit. J Neurosurg Anesthesiol 2001;13:163–75.
116. Dalessio DJ. Current concepts. Seizure disorders and pregnancy. N Engl J Med 1985;312:559–63.
117. Raps EC, Galetta SL, Flamm ES. Neuro-intensive care of the pregnant woman. Neurol Clin 1994;12:601–11.
118. Goetting MG, Davidson BN. Status epilepticus during labor. A case report. J Reprod Med 1987;32:313–4.
119. Ryan G, Lange IR, Naugler MA. Clinical experience with phenytoin prophylaxis in severe preeclampsia. Am J Obstet Gynecol 1989;161:1297–304.
120. Spike J. Brain death, pregnancy, and posthumous motherhood. J Clin Ethics 1999;10:57–65.
121. Esmaeilzadeh M, Dictus C, Kayvanpour E, et al. One life ends, another begins: management of a brain-dead pregnant mother–A systematic review. BMC Med 2010;8:74.
122. Bernstein IM, Watson M, Simmons GM, et al. Maternal brain death and prolonged fetal survival. Obstet Gynecol 1989;74:434–7.
123. Mallampalli A, Guy E. Cardiac arrest in pregnancy and somatic support after brain death. Crit Care Med 2005;33:S325–31.
124. Varelas P, Fayad P. Migraine and stroke. In: Cohen S, editor. Management of ischemic stroke. 1st edition. McGraw-Hill; 2000. p. 391–404.
125. Bodis L, Szupera Z, Pierantozzi M, et al. Neurological complications of pregnancy. J Neurol Sci 1998;153:279–93.

Liver Failure in Pregnancy

Stephen J. Bacak, DO, MPH, Loralei L. Thornburg, MD*

KEYWORDS

- Pregnancy • Liver failure • Acute fatty liver of pregnancy • HELLP syndrome
- Viral infections

KEY POINTS

- Acute liver failure in pregnancy should be evaluated for both pregnancy-related and non–pregnancy-related causes.
- Acute fatty liver of pregnancy is rare but has a high maternal and fetal mortality rate, so acute liver failure in pregnancy should include evaluation for this disorder.
- HELLP (hemolysis, elevated liver enzymes, low platelet) syndrome occurs in less than 1% of all pregnancies but may be seen in up to 20% of pregnancies complicated by pre-eclampsia, and can lead to acute liver failure especially with associated liver hematomas or liver rupture.
- Therapy should be similar to that for the nonpregnant patient, and no life-saving intervention should be withheld from a patient with acute liver failure in pregnancy.

INTRODUCTION

Acute liver failure (ALF), also known as fulminant hepatic failure, is an uncommon but life-threatening condition[1] caused by an acute hepatic insult or injury with subsequent development of encephalopathy and coagulopathy.[1–3] The underlying hepatic cell necrosis, apoptosis, and inflammatory response may precipitate multiorgan failure.[4] ALF can further be broken down into hyperacute (0–1 weeks), acute (1–4 weeks), and subacute (4–12 weeks) phases according to the onset of symptoms and development of encephalopathy.[1,5] Although severe liver disease and ALF are rare, there is still an estimated worldwide incidence of 1 to 10 cases per million persons per year.[1,2] Survival rates have increased in the last decade because of improved understanding of the underlying disease processes and advances in critical care. Although ALF in pregnancy is extremely rare, the outcomes, both maternal and fetal, can be devastating. It is estimated that liver disease occurs in approximately 3% of pregnancies, although the true incidence of ALF in pregnancy is unknown. Most often, pregnancy-related diseases

Authorship Disclosures: None.

Division of Maternal-Fetal Medicine, University of Rochester Medical Center, 601 Elmwood Avenue, Box 668, Rochester, NY 14642, USA

* Corresponding author.

E-mail address: Loralei_Thornburg@urmc.rochester.edu

such as acute fatty liver of pregnancy (AFLP) and hemolysis, elevated liver enzymes, and low platelet (HELLP) syndrome are the origin of liver failure in pregnancy.

This review provides an overview of the normal liver changes that occur during pregnancy, and describes the most common conditions of ALF and general management strategies of ALF during pregnancy. Preeclampsia and eclampsia are discussed in detail in separate reviews.

NORMAL LIVER FUNCTION DURING PREGNANCY

Despite increases in cardiac output, blood flow to the liver remains essentially unchanged (approximately 25%–33% of cardiac output) during pregnancy.[6,7] The liver may be slightly elevated within the abdomen with increasing gestation, owing to displacement by the enlarging uterus.[8] However, hepatomegaly is abnormal and should prompt an immediate evaluation of underlying liver disease. Liver enzymes including alanine aminotransferase (ALT), aspartate aminotransferase (AST), γ-glutamyl transferase (GGT), and bilirubin remain normal or may decrease about 20% in pregnancy compared with the nonpregnant patient.[6,7] Alkaline phosphatase (ALP) increases with advancing gestation as a result of placental production, and high levels should not be considered abnormal. Total protein decreases during pregnancy, primarily because of a decrease in serum albumin. Increased levels of estrogen cause an increase in fibrinogen and other clotting factors (factors VII, VIII, IX, and X).[9] Ceruloplasmin and transferrin are also elevated during pregnancy.

Suspicions for a pathologic process should be raised with elevations in liver markers during pregnancy. In general, elevations in ALT, a more specific liver marker, and AST are caused by hepatocyte necrosis after injury and enzyme release into the circulation.[6] However, while minor elevations may suggest liver disease, slight elevations (less than 1.5 times the upper limit of normal) in ALT and AST may also represent normal distribution.[6] These values are also known to be higher in obese individuals and a small number of people with a defect in enzyme clearance.

PREGNANCY-RELATED CAUSES OF LIVER FAILURE
Acute Fatty Liver of Pregnancy

AFLP occurs in 1 of 7000 to 16,000 pregnancies, primarily in the third trimester (**Table 1**).[7,10] The incidence is higher in primigravid women, multiple gestations, and pregnancies with a male fetus. The exact pathophysiology is unknown. It is thought that AFLP is caused by microvesicular fatty infiltration of the hepatocytes.[10] More specifically, recent data suggest the defects in long-chain fatty acid oxidation attributable to a deficiency in the enzyme long-chain 3-hydroxyacyl coenzyme A dehydrogenase (LCHAD) in fetal mitochondria result in accumulation of fatty acids in the maternal circulation and hepatocytes.[11,12] This accumulation results in hepatotoxicity and eventually leads to liver failure. Though rare, the maternal and neonatal mortality rates are high, up to 18% and 55%, respectively.[10] Sixteen cases of AFLP were identified in a 10-year review from 3 tertiary care centers.[10] The majority, 69%, of patients developed AFLP during pregnancy, with the remaining cases identified within 4 postpartum days. In this review, 12.5% of the patients died and there were 3 fetal deaths. Pereira and colleagues[13] found a similar mortality rate in their 10-year single-institution review. In a large retrospective study from the Netherlands, the maternal mortality ratio from AFLP was 0.13 per 100,000 births, and the incidence of severe maternal morbidity (including admission to intensive care unit, uterine rupture, eclampsia/HELLP syndrome with liver hematoma, and hemorrhage requiring transfusion) was 3.2 per 100,000 deliveries.[14]

Table 1
Clinical features and laboratory findings in common underlying conditions of acute liver failure during pregnancy

	HELLP	AFLP	Viral Hepatitis
Risk factors	Prior pregnancy with HELLP Multiple gestation Extremes of age	Primigravida Multiple gestation Male fetus	Same as nonpregnant (blood, fecal/oral transmission depending on type)
Typical gestational age of onset	>20 wk	>24 wk	Any, evenly distributed through trimesters
Prior/family history?			
Typical clinical features	Hemolysis Thrombocytopenia Elevated liver function tests With/without hypertension With/without proteinuria DIC and liver failure (rare)	Liver failure Coagulopathy Encephalopathy Hyperammonemia Hypoglycemia DIC Jaundice	Liver failure Coagulopathy Encephalopathy DIC — — —
Diagnosis			
AST/ALT levels	Mild, up to 20× normal	300–500 IU/L but may vary	>1000 IU/L
Bilirubin	<5 mg/dL	<5 mg/dL but may be higher	Variable
Imaging	Normal in most, infarcts, hematomas, capsular rupture (rare)	Fatty infiltration	Normal
Outcomes			
Maternal mortality	1%	7%–18%	41%–54% (hepatitis E)
Fetal/perinatal mortality	11% (gestational age dependent)	9%–23% (gestational age dependent)	69% (hepatitis E) 39% (HSV)
Recurrence	25%, aspirin therapy starting at 16 wk may decrease risk	High if LCHAD deficiency, otherwise rare	None

Abbreviations: ALT, alanine aminotransferase; AST, aspartate aminotransferase; DIC, disseminated intravascular coagulation; HELLP, hemolysis/elevated liver enzymes/low platelet syndrome; HSV, herpes simplex virus; LCHAD, long-chain 3-hydroxyacyl coenzyme A dehydrogenase.

Adapted from Shams M. Update in liver diseases with pregnancy. Gastroenterology and Hepatology Research 2013;2(2):393.

The clinical presentation of AFLP varies. Nausea, vomiting, and epigastric pain are the most common symptoms.[7,11,15] Other symptoms include jaundice, anorexia, malaise, hypertension, headache, pulmonary edema, multiorgan failure, pancreatitis, disseminated intravascular coagulation (DIC), and proteinuria. AFLP and HELLP are coexistent in approximately 50% of patients.[9] Diagnostic criteria include moderate elevations in ALT and AST. Bilirubin, blood urea nitrogen, uric acid, and creatinine are also mildly elevated.[10] Hypoglycemia is common, and often the distinguishing factor in differentiating from preeclampsia and HELLP syndrome and making an accurate diagnosis. However, the absence of hypoglycemia should not rule out the disease, as this can be an absent or a late finding in AFLP. DIC is also often present in late disease. A liver biopsy can confirm the diagnosis of AFLP, although a biopsy is rarely obtained because of the risks to the severely ill patient with coagulopathy. Immediate delivery and prompt resuscitation are vital to the survival of both the mother and fetus. The fetus should be tested for LCHAD deficiency through newborn screening.

Hemolysis, Elevated Liver Enzymes, Low Platelet Syndrome

HELLP syndrome falls within the spectrum of hypertensive disorders of pregnancy, and is most closely associated with preeclampsia with severe features (see **Table 1**).[16] (As of 2013, the terms "preeclampsia" and "preeclampsia with severe features" have replaced the less precise "mild preeclampsia" and "severe preeclampsia.")[17] HELLP syndrome occurs in less than 1% of all pregnancies but may be seen in up to 20% of pregnancies complicated by preeclampsia with severe features. HELLP syndrome occurs both in the antepartum (two-thirds of cases) and postpartum periods (one-third of cases).[16,17] Risk factors mimic those for preeclampsia and include white race, very young and advanced maternal age, multiple gestation, multiparous women, and prior history of preeclampsia or HELLP syndrome.[11]

Though not entirely understood, the pathogenesis of HELLP syndrome is thought to be similar to preeclampsia, and involves abnormal development of the placenta and endothelial dysfunction.[18] Specific physiologic processes include activation of the complement and coagulation cascade systems, vascular injury and inflammation, and fibrin deposition. The vasoconstriction, increase in vascular tone, and platelet aggregation that occurs eventually results in thrombocytopenia and hepatocellular necrosis. Pregnant women with HELLP syndrome will often present with vague complaints of right upper quadrant pain, epigastric pain, and nausea and/or vomiting. Hypertension is common but may be absent in 15% to 20% of cases.[19] Some women will also complain of neurologic symptoms such as headaches and visual disturbances, similarly to preeclampsia with severe features. Significant complications include DIC, placental abruption, acute renal failure, pulmonary edema, retinal detachment, liver hematomas, liver rupture, and ALF.[16,19,20] The risk of maternal death in HELLP syndrome is approximately 1%.[16]

Acute Hepatic Rupture

Hepatic rupture occurs in approximately 1% of women diagnosed with HELLP syndrome. However, if it occurs there is a substantial risk of ALF and both maternal and fetal mortality.[11] Although liver rupture is associated with HELLP and preeclampsia in most cases, rupture has been reported in other conditions such as focal nodular hyperplasia.[21] The underlying pathophysiology is unknown, but studies have suggested that fibrin deposition in intrahepatic sinusoids may play a role. This deposition leads to an obstruction and eventual capsule rupture, thrombi formation, and tissue necrosis.[8] Liver rupture resulting from subcapsular hematomas are usually located on the right lobe of the liver. As expected, patients present with right upper quadrant or lower chest pain secondary to irritation of the liver capsule.[11] With further stretching and capsule rupture, patients experience significant abdominal pain, distention, and signs of hypovolemic and hemorrhagic shock. If the hematoma remains unruptured and the woman is hemodynamically stable, conservative management and supportive care are recommended. Suspicion for rupture requires immediate delivery and surgical exploration, given the high maternal and fetal mortality rates.

PREEXISTING OR UNRELATED CAUSES OF LIVER FAILURE DURING PREGNANCY
Acetaminophen and Toxic Overdose

Acetaminophen toxicity is the most common cause of ALF in the United States, accounting for approximately 42% of all cases.[22,23] Unintentional acetaminophen overdose accounts for most cases. Data from the Acute Liver Failure Study Group suggest the incidence in the United States is increasing.[23,24] In pregnancy, acetaminophen is routinely used and generally considered safe. However, acetaminophen overdose is fairly common in pregnancy. Patients exceeding 4 g per day are at risk for hepatotoxicity.[22] Most of the acetaminophen is metabolized in the liver to nontoxic products after conjugation with glucuronide or sulfate before urine excretion. However, a small portion of acetaminophen is metabolized into the more toxic metabolite N-acetyl-p-benzoquinoneimine, which during an acute overdose or chronic ingestion may cause pericentral necrosis and hepatocyte death.[22,25] Nausea and vomiting are commonly cited symptoms during an acetaminophen overdose, and after ingestion of large doses a person may present with metabolic acidosis, coagulopathy, acute renal failure, pancreatitis, and coma. However, some patients may have no symptoms before the onset of liver failure. Acetaminophen is also known to readily cross the placenta, and overdose may lead to fetal liver injury and even death, with the greatest risk occurring in the third trimester. Acetaminophen levels should not be checked for at least 4 hours after ingestion, and transaminitis usually peaks after 72 hours.[25] Franko and colleagues[26] published the first case of hepatic failure secondary to acetaminophen overdose that resulted in the patient receiving a liver transplant. In a case report by Thornton and Minns,[27] chronic and excessive use of acetaminophen during pregnancy led to liver failure requiring transplant and fetal demise.

Overall, more than 1100 drugs (including antibiotics, salicylates, selective serotonin reuptake inhibitors, herbal remedies, vitamins, and supplements) have been linked to liver injury and failure.[28] The data regarding these medications, overdosing, and ALF during pregnancy are limited. A high clinical suspicion is warranted in making an accurate diagnosis, and appropriate therapy should be administered to the patient regardless of pregnancy status.

Viral Infections

Viral infections remain a well-known cause of liver failure during pregnancy. Worldwide, hepatitis infections are responsible for most cases of AFL.[1] Hepatitis A, B, and C have the same frequency in pregnant women as in the nonpregnant population, and the onset is equally distributed throughout the trimesters (see **Table 1**). Although all hepatitis strains can cause failure in pregnancy, hepatitis E virus (HEV) is of particular concern. HEV is a single-stranded RNA virus that is common in developing countries and transmitted through a fecal-oral route. The incubation period ranges from 2 to 9 weeks. Unlike hepatitis B (HBV) and hepatitis C (HCV) viruses, HEV does not progress to a chronic state. Outside of pregnancy, HEV infection is mild. However, pregnant women with acute HEV infection are at risk for fulminant hepatitis, liver failure, and high maternal mortality and morbidity rates.[7,29] In an attempt to identify causes associated with this high mortality rate of HEV, Borkakoti and colleagues[29] found that the viral loads of HEV in pregnant women with ALF were significantly higher than those in nonpregnant women.

Fulminant herpes simplex virus (HSV) hepatitis has been reported in the literature.[30–32] Similar to pregnancy-related causes of liver failure, HSV hepatitis typically presents in the third trimester and is thought to be due to the immunocompromised state of pregnancy.[31] HSV-1 and HSV-2 serotypes, and both primary and secondary infections, have been reported in HSV hepatitis.[32] Maternal mortality rates are high, approaching 40%. Antiviral therapy with acyclovir is considered the first line of treatment. However, a recent case report highlights the concern for antiviral-resistant disease.[30]

Acute on Chronic Liver Failure

Acute on chronic liver failure (ACLF) describes ALF in patients with underlying cirrhosis or conditions secondary to a new hepatic insult or further deterioration in liver dysfunction.[33,34] In ACLF there is a rapid decline in liver function and a high mortality rate, approaching 90% in some cases. The underlying inflammatory or infectious processes exacerbating liver damage also lead to deterioration in renal function, encephalopathy, coagulation disorders, and cardiac dysfunction.[34] Pregnancy in women with chronic liver disease is rare, although the prevalence may be increasing with the increase in advanced maternal age and the use of assisted reproductive technology.

Budd-Chiari syndrome (BCS) results from an outflow obstruction of the hepatic veins and is commonly associated with the use of estrogen-containing oral contraceptives. However, pregnancy has been reported in 16% of patients with BCS.[7,35] The increased prothrombotic state of pregnancy may exacerbate the underlying condition. Favorable pregnancy outcomes in the setting of BCS have been reported.[35,36] Clinically, women present with right upper quadrant pain, abdominal distention, nausea and vomiting, jaundice, and ascites. Some women with significant venous obstruction may rapidly deteriorate secondary to portal hypertension, variceal bleeding, and fulminant liver failure requiring portal caval shunting or even transplantation. Diagnosis should include an evaluation of coexisting thrombophilias including factor V Leiden, antithrombin III deficiency, and antiphospholipid antibodies.[37,38] Polycythemia vera is also associated with BCS.

Cirrhosis is an irreversible disease of the liver that ultimately leads to end-stage liver failure secondary to chronic hepatocellular fibrosis and destruction.[39] As a result, portal hypertension develops and substantially increases the risk of morbidity during pregnancy. There have been several reports of pregnancy in women with cirrhosis, and improvements in the management of cirrhosis have led to favorable maternal and neonatal outcomes in these women. However, pregnancy still poses an increased risk for morbidity and mortality caused by worsening portal hypertension, hemorrhage, splenic artery aneurysm, and liver failure.[40] Mortality rates are thought to be as high as 10% to 18%.

MANAGEMENT
Acute Liver Failure

Optimal management of ALF in pregnancy begins with early recognition and accurate diagnosis of the underlying etiology. In ideal circumstances, a coordinated multidisciplinary effort should take place that includes critical care specialists, maternal-fetal medicine physicians, hepatologists or gastroenterologists, neonatologists, and surgical transplant teams. The physiologic and anatomic changes that occur during pregnancy may provide diagnostic challenges for ALF; however, as pregnancy itself is rarely a cause of ALF, other possible causes should be thoroughly evaluated. Furthermore, there are few evidence-based recommendations for managing the pregnant woman with ALF. Therefore, management of ALF should be guided by the same principles followed for the nonpregnant patient.

Recommended laboratory chemistries are shown in **Box 1**. Although ultrasonography serves as the gold standard for imaging in pregnancy because of its safety

Box 1
Recommended laboratory tests in the diagnosis and management of acute liver failure during pregnancy

Hematology

    Complete blood count

    Type and screen

    PT

    aPTT

    INR

    Lactate

Serum Chemistry

    Electrolytes

    Liver function tests (ALT, AST, GGT, bilirubin, albumin)

    Amylase

    Lipase

Arterial Blood Gas

    Lactate

    Ammonia

Toxicology Screen

    Acetaminophen

    Cocaine

    Alcohol

Autoimmune

    ANA

    Anti–smooth muscle antibody

    Microsomal antibodies

Hepatitis Serology

    Anti-HAV IgM

    HBsAg

    Anti-HBc IgM

    Antihepatitis E

Additional Viral Serology

    CMV

    EBV

    HSV

    HIV

Other

    Ceruloplasmin

    Serum copper

Abbreviations: ALT, alanine aminotransferase; ANA, antinuclear antibody; aPTT, activated partial thromboplastin time; AST, aspartate aminotransferase; CMV, cytomegalovirus; EBV, Epstein-Barr virus; GGT, γ-glutamyl transferase; HAV, hepatitis A virus; HBc, hepatitis B core; HBsAg, hepatitis B surface antigen; HIV, human immunodeficiency virus; HSV, herpes simplex virus; IgM, immunoglobulin M; INR, international normalized ratio; PT, prothrombin time.

profile, computed tomography (CT) and MRI should be considered to further characterize the liver.[41] One advantage of MRI is that there is no radiation exposure to the mother or fetus. Gadolinium contrast is relatively contraindicated in pregnancy because of the theoretic concern of concentration within the fetal cavity. However, depending on the availability of an MRI-trained radiologist and the acuity of the situation, a CT of the abdomen and pelvis with appropriate shielding of the fetus, if possible, may provide quicker results. No imaging should be withheld in pregnancy if clinically indicated, especially if it will alter management or aid in diagnosis, as delay in diagnosis and management can substantially worsen outcomes for both mother and fetus. A liver biopsy may provide valuable histologic information and influence the timing of delivery, and should be considered if the patient is hemodynamically stable.

For most patients, the management and recommended treatment is similar between both pregnant and nonpregnant patients. Avoidance of further liver-toxic agents in combination with supportive care is the typical therapy, as liver recovery for most patients with a self-limited cause resulting in ALF is the gold standard. For those patients in whom the evaluation suggests pregnancy-related ALF (eg, AFLP, severe HELLP), delivery is recommended (if possible after antenatal corticosteroids for fetal lung maturity are administered) to facilitate recovery and improve both maternal and fetal outcomes. If the diagnosis is unclear, as many of the clinical features and laboratory evaluations of these conditions overlap, and AFLP or HELLP are the leading diagnoses, delivery and subsequent recovery from ALF may allow establishment of a definitive diagnosis. No therapy that is considered life-saving or standard of care for ALF should be withheld simply for reasons of pregnancy status, as the risks of untreated or fulminant ALF are generally higher than the fetal risk from therapy. In addition, the risk of poor fetal outcome for those patients with ALF in the first and second trimester (before viability) is so high that maternal survival and concerns should take precedence, and pregnancy termination should be strongly considered. A maternal-fetal medicine physician and a toxicologist can help to advise on the risks of specific therapies in pregnancy, but for most patients the maternal and fetal benefit of liver recovery outweigh most potential risks.

Similarly, the course, presentation, and management of viral hepatitis are the same as for nonpregnant patients. Viral hepatitis is typically not a reason for delivery, termination, or cesarean section. Breastfeeding is safe and should be encouraged. Unless transplantation is required, care is typically supportive.

Chronic Liver Failure

There are considerable risks for those patients with chronic liver failure, regardless of cause, entering pregnancy. Patients' underlying disease should be optimally controlled and stable on medications for several months before conception. Medications should be adjusted to minimize pregnancy risks. Safety profiles of commonly used medications in the management of chronic liver disease during pregnancy are shown in **Table 2**. Vitamin K therapy should be established if needed. For those patients with cirrhotic liver disease before pregnancy, prepregnancy endoscopy to establish the presence and extent of varicosities, and treatment of those that are amenable to therapy, is ideal. Should the patient with chronic liver failure become pregnant, evaluation and treatment in the first trimester can also be safely accomplished. Those with prior thrombosis should maintain recommended anticoagulation but should change from warfarin to low molecular weight heparin before conception. Women on chronic aspirin therapy should continue their recommended daily doses. For women not on chronic aspirin therapy, especially those with a history of

Table 2 Safety profile for common medications used for chronic liver disease during pregnancy	
Drug	**Uses and Safety**
Adefovir	Limited data, maternal nephrotoxicity and lactic acidosis
Azathioprine	Low risk, increased risk for spontaneous abortion and congenital malformations
β-Blockers	Low risk, slightly increased risk for intrauterine growth restriction
Cyclosporine	Probably safe, immunosuppression
Entecavir	Limited data, maternal lactic acidosis
Hydroxyzine	Probably safe, risk of neonatal withdrawal syndrome
Interferon	Generally not recommended, case reports of intrauterine growth restriction
Lamivudine	Low risk, no known teratogenicity
Mycophenolate mofetil	Contraindicated, fetal facial anomalies
Octreotide	Probably safe, no known teratogenicity
Penicillamine	Therapy for Wilson disease. Risk of agranulocytosis but should be maintained to prevent liver deterioration
Prednisone	Low risk, slightly increased risk of cleft lip in first trimester, increased risk of gestational diabetes
Ribavirin	Contraindicated because of fetal embryopathy
Tacrolimus	Probably safe
Ursodeoxycholic acid	Low risk
Vasopressin	Avoid because of increased risk of uterine ischemia

Adapted from Tan J, Surti B, Saab S. Pregnancy and cirrhosis. Liver Transpl 2008;14(8):1084–5; and Shams M. Update in liver diseases with pregnancy. Gastroenterology and Hepatology Research 2013;2(2):396.

preeclampsia with severe features or HELLP syndrome, this should be considered given the association between low-dose aspirin and a decreased risk for recurrent preeclampsia.[17] Aspirin also offers some preventive benefit to the increased risk for thrombosis during pregnancy. In patients with chronic liver disease and associated splenomegaly and thrombocytopenia resulting from sequestration, prepregnancy splenectomy can improve platelet counts. However, this decision, if needed during pregnancy, should be made jointly with maternal-fetal medicine and liver failure specialists. Platelet counts are expected to worsen slightly throughout pregnancy, and therefore should be followed closely.

Transplantation

Liver transplantation has become the gold standard for treatment of both acute and chronic liver failure, and has led to significant improvements in mortality and long-term morbidity. It is difficult to predict which patients will require liver transplantation among those with AFL during pregnancy. Similar to other diseases of pregnancy, resolution after delivery is common. Therefore, delivery and supportive care may improve liver function and allow avoidance of transplant. For the patient with ALF that becomes advanced or the chronic liver failure patient in whom further liver decompensation occurs, a liver transplant may be recommended. However, evaluation and determination of the need for liver transplantation is generally made according to criteria similar to those for the nonpregnant patient. Delivery before transplant is likely to be recommended regardless of gestational age, as fetal loss during liver transplantation is high.

Pregnancy after transplantation is generally well tolerated and has favorable outcomes.[42–45] Vernadakis and colleagues[46] also reported on a successful orthotopic liver transplant that took place hours after a 34-week cesarean delivery in a woman with hepatic failure secondary to acute hepatitis B infection. At present there is no recommendation for the optimal timing of pregnancy after liver transplantation. Many transplant centers recommend delaying pregnancy for at least 1 year after transplantation, whereas others have advocated for extended interval periods.[47,48] The risk of rejection during pregnancy seems minimal if the transplant is stable at the time of conception. Some studies report an increased rate of pregnancy-related hypertension, but others have not found such a relationship.[42,43,49,50] The use of immunosuppressive agents has been shown to be beneficial in gravid liver transplant patients.[44,51] Patients should be on stable doses of commonly used immunosuppressants with known risks and safety profiles during pregnancy.

SUMMARY

ALF in pregnancy is rare, but the potential for fetal loss and maternal morbidity and mortality is high. When encountering ALF in pregnancy, the clinician must evaluate for both pregnancy-related and non–pregnancy-related causes. No therapy that is considered life-saving should be withheld from a patient with ALF in pregnancy. For those women with pregnancy-related liver failure, delivery may allow for quicker recovery and improved survival of both the mother and infant.

REFERENCES

1. Bernal W, Wendon J. Acute liver failure. N Engl J Med 2013;369(26):2525–34.
2. Bernal W, Auzinger G, Dhawan A, et al. Acute liver failure. Lancet 2010; 376(9736):190–201.
3. Lee WM, Stravitz RT, Larson AM. Introduction to the revised American Association for the Study of Liver Diseases position paper on acute liver failure 2011. Hepatology 2012;55(3):965–7.
4. Willars C. Update in intensive care medicine: acute liver failure. Initial management, supportive treatment and who to transplant. Curr Opin Crit Care 2014; 20(2):202–9.
5. O'Grady JG, Schalm SW, Williams R. Acute liver failure: redefining the syndromes. Lancet 1993;342(8866):273–5.
6. Jamjute P, Ahmad A, Ghosh T, et al. Liver function test and pregnancy. J Matern Fetal Neonatal Med 2009;22(3):274–83.
7. Joshi D, James A, Quaglia A, et al. Liver disease in pregnancy. Lancet 2010; 375(9714):594–605.
8. Guntupalli SR, Steingrub J. Hepatic disease and pregnancy: an overview of diagnosis and management. Crit Care Med 2005;33(Supplement):S332–9.
9. Williamson C. Diseases of the liver, biliary system, and pancreas. Creasy and Resnik's maternal-fetal medicine: principles and practice. 7th edition. Philadelphia: Elsevier; 2014.
10. Fesenmeier MF, Coppage KH, Lambers DS, et al. Acute fatty liver of pregnancy in 3 tertiary care centers. Am J Obstet Gynecol 2005;192(5):1416–9.
11. Schutt VA, Minuk GY. Liver diseases unique to pregnancy. Best Pract Res Clin Gastroenterol 2007;21(5):771–92.

12. McNulty J. Acute fatty liver of pregnancy. Obstetric intensive care manual. 3rd edition. New York: The McGraw-Hill Companies, Inc; 2011. p. 183–90.

13. Pereira SP, O'Donohue J, Wendon J, et al. Maternal and perinatal outcome in severe pregnancy-related liver disease. Hepatology 1997;26(5):1258–62.

14. Dekker RR, Schutte JM, Stekelenburg J, et al. Maternal mortality and severe maternal morbidity from acute fatty liver of pregnancy in the Netherlands. Eur J Obstet Gynecol Reprod Biol 2011;157(1):27–31.

15. Chen H, Yuan L, Tan J, et al. Severe liver disease in pregnancy. Int J Gynaecol Obstet 2008;101(3):277–80.

16. Sibai BM, Ramadan MK, Usta I, et al. Maternal morbidity and mortality in 442 pregnancies with hemolysis, elevated liver enzymes, and low platelets (HELLP syndrome). Am J Obstet Gynecol 1993;169(4):1000–6.

17. American College of Obstetricians and Gynecologists. Hypertension in pregnancy. Report of the American College of Obstetricians and Gynecologists' task force on hypertension in pregnancy. Obstet Gynecol 2013;122(5):1122–31.

18. Rahman TM, Wendon J. Severe hepatic dysfunction in pregnancy. QJM 2002;95: 343–57.

19. Sibai BM. Diagnosis, controversies, and management of the syndrome of hemolysis, elevated liver enzymes, and low platelet count. Obstet Gynecol 2004;103(5 Pt 1): 981–91.

20. Shames BD, Fernandez LA, Sollinger HW, et al. Liver transplantation for HELLP syndrome. Liver Transpl 2005;11(2):224–8.

21. Yajima D, Kondo F, Nakatani Y, et al. A fatal case of subcapsular liver hemorrhage in late pregnancy: a review of hemorrhages caused by hepatocellular hyperplastic nodules. J Forensic Sci 2013;58(Suppl 1):S253–7.

22. Fontana RJ. Acute liver failure including acetaminophen overdose. Med Clin North Am 2008;92(4):761–94.

23. Larson AM, Polson J, Fontana RJ, et al. Acetaminophen-induced acute liver failure: results of a United States multicenter, prospective study. Hepatology 2005; 42(6):1364–72.

24. Ostapowicz G, Fontana RJ, Schiodt FV, et al. Results of a prospective study of acute liver failure at 17 tertiary care centers in the United States. Ann Intern Med 2002;137(12):947–54.

25. Gei AF, Suarez V. Poisoning in pregnancy. Obstetric intensive care manual. 3rd edition. 2011. p. 275–88.

26. Franko KR, Mekeel KL, Woelkers D, et al. Accidental acetaminophen overdose results in liver transplant during second trimester of pregnancy: a case report. Transplant Proc 2013;45(5):2063–5.

27. Thornton SL, Minns AB. Unintentional chronic acetaminophen poisoning during pregnancy resulting in liver transplantation. J Med Toxicol 2012;8(2): 176–8.

28. Reuben A, Koch DG, Lee WM, Acute Liver Failure Study Group. Drug-induced acute liver failure: results of a U.S. multicenter, prospective study. Hepatology 2010;52(6):2065–76.

29. Borkakoti J, Hazam RK, Mohammad A, et al. Does high viral load of hepatitis E virus influence the severity and prognosis of acute liver failure during pregnancy? J Med Virol 2013;85(4):620–6.

30. Herrera CA, Eichelberger KY, Chescheir NC. Antiviral-resistant fulminant herpes hepatitis in pregnancy. AJP Rep 2013;3(2):87–90.

31. Kang AH, Graves CR. Herpes simplex hepatitis in pregnancy: a case report and review of the literature. Obstet Gynecol Surv 1999;54(7):463–8.

32. Allen RH, Tuomala RE. Herpes simplex virus hepatitis causing acute liver dysfunction and thrombocytopenia in pregnancy. Obstet Gynecol 2005;106(5 Pt 2): 1187–9.
33. Jalan R, Gines P, Olson JC, et al. Acute-on chronic liver failure. J Hepatol 2012; 57(6):1336–48.
34. Vizzutti F, Arena U, Laffi G, et al. Acute on chronic liver failure: from pathophysiology to clinical management. Trends Anaesth Crit Care 2013;3(3):122–9.
35. Rautou PE, Angermayr B, Garcia-Pagan JC, et al. Pregnancy in women with known and treated Budd-Chiari syndrome: maternal and fetal outcomes. J Hepatol 2009; 51(1):47–54.
36. Aggarwal N, Suri V, Chopra S, et al. Pregnancy outcome in Budd Chiari Syndrome—a tertiary care centre experience. Arch Gynecol Obstet 2013;288(4): 949–52.
37. Fickert P, Ramschak H, Kenner L, et al. Acute Budd-Chiari syndrome with fulminant hepatic failure in a pregnant woman with factor V Leiden mutation. Gastroenterology 1996;111(6):1670–3.
38. Segal S, Shenhav S, Segal O, et al. Budd-Chiari syndrome complicating severe preeclampsia in a parturient with primary antiphospholipid syndrome. Eur J Obstet Gynecol Reprod Biol 1996;68(1–2):227–9.
39. Russell MA, Craigo SD. Cirrhosis and portal hypertension in pregnancy. Semin Perinatol 1998;22(2):156–65.
40. Tan J, Surti B, Saab S. Pregnancy and cirrhosis. Liver Transpl 2008;14(8):1081–91.
41. Hodnett PA, Maher MM. Imaging of gastrointestinal and hepatic diseases during pregnancy. Best Pract Res Clin Gastroenterol 2007;21(5):901–17.
42. Dei Malatesta MF, Rossi M, Rocca B, et al. Pregnancy after liver transplantation: report of 8 new cases and review of the literature. Transpl Immunol 2006;15(4): 297–302.
43. Jabiry-Zieniewicz Z, Cyganek A, Luterek K, et al. Pregnancy and delivery after liver transplantation. Transplant Proc 2005;37(2):1197–200.
44. Jabiry-Zieniewicz Z, Kaminski P, Pietrzak B, et al. Outcome of four high-risk pregnancies in female liver transplant recipients on tacrolimus immunosuppression. Transplant Proc 2006;38(1):255–7.
45. Kociszewska-Najman B, Pietrzak B, Jabiry-Zieniewicz Z, et al. Pregnancy after living related liver transplantation—a report of two cases. Ann Transplant 2012; 17(3):120–5.
46. Vernadakis S, Fouzas I, Kykalos S, et al. Successful salvage delivery and liver transplantation for fulminant hepatic failure in a 34-week pregnant woman: a case report. Transplant Proc 2012;44(9):2768–9.
47. Bonanno C, Dove L. Pregnancy after liver transplantation. Semin Perinatol 2007; 31(6):348–53.
48. Nagy S, Bush MC, Berkowitz R, et al. Pregnancy outcome in liver transplant recipients. Obstet Gynecol 2003;102(1):121–8.
49. Coffin CS, Shaheen AA, Burak KW, et al. Pregnancy outcomes among liver transplant recipients in the United States: a nationwide case-control analysis. Liver Transpl 2010;16(1):56–63.
50. Deshpande NA, James NT, Kucirka LM, et al. Pregnancy outcomes of liver transplant recipients: a systematic review and meta-analysis. Liver Transpl 2012;18(6):621–9.
51. Alvaro E, Jimenez LC, Palomo I, et al. Pregnancy and orthotopic liver transplantation. Transplant Proc 2013;45(5):1966–8.

Renal Failure in Pregnancy

Ari Balofsky, MD, Maksim Fedarau, MD*

KEYWORDS

- Renal failure • Pregnancy • Preeclampsia • HELLP • Thrombotic microangiopathies
- Acute fatty liver of pregnancy • Dialysis

KEY POINTS

- Renal failure in pregnancy is a rare but severe complication that can have significant long-term effects on both mother and fetus.
- Evaluation of the pregnant patient must take into consideration normal physiologic changes of pregnancy that increase the complexity of diagnosing renal failure.
- The etiology of renal failure in the pregnant patient is divided into prerenal, intrarenal, and postrenal causes; treatment focuses on the underlying cause.
- Supportive measures such as fluid resuscitation are the basis of treatment for renal failure in pregnancy, with delivery usually being the ultimate goal.
- When other measures fail dialysis may be required, with the goal of prolonging pregnancy until delivery becomes feasible, and providing an environment suitable for fetal growth.

INTRODUCTION

Renal failure is a potentially devastating complication during pregnancy that can affect both mother and fetus. It may be related to preexisting renal disease, or may develop as a new entity during pregnancy. Preexisting chronic renal disease occurs in about 4% of parturients. These women have a 43% increased risk of pregnancy-related renal dysfunction, and 10% of patients will develop a rapid deterioration of renal function.[1,2] Acute renal failure (ARF) presents an important clinical challenge and, although rare, it can be associated with significant morbidity and mortality. In the nonpregnant patient, ARF has been defined by various changes including serum creatinine increased by 0.5 mg/dL or greater over baseline, or a greater than 50% increase over baseline, or a 50% reduction in creatinine clearance, or renal dysfunction requiring dialysis.[3] Oliguria is often seen with ARF in pregnant patients, defined as urine output of less than 0.5 mL/kg/h. Although this definition has been standardized for the nonpregnant patient by the Risk–Injury–Failure–Loss–End (RIFLE) classification

The authors have nothing to disclose.
Department of Anesthesiology, University of Rochester Medical Center, 601 Elmwood, Box 604, Rochester, NY 14642, USA
* Corresponding author.
E-mail address: Maksim_Fedarau@URMC.Rochester.edu

system,[4] no such standard definition exists for the parturient, although Mantel[5] has used a clinical definition of oliguria of less than 400 mL per 24 hours not responsive to therapy, or an acute increase in serum urea to greater than 15 mmol/L or creatinine of greater than 400 mol/L. The incidence of ARF has decreased from 1/3000 to 1/15,000 to 1/20,000 since the 1960s, mainly owing to improved prenatal care and decreases in septic complications, such as abortions. Despite the decrease in incidence, overall mortality rates have remained in the 0% to 30% range, and the long-term prognosis has also remained consistent, with full recovery rates of 60% to 90% after episodes of ARF.[2] To effectively evaluate and treat the pregnant patient with renal failure, the underlying etiology must be identified correctly.

PATIENT EVALUATION OVERVIEW

Evaluating renal failure in the parturient can be a complex task, especially given the lack of a commonly accepted definition of the condition. Many different factors must be considered, including the normal physiologic changes of pregnancy and the variety of conditions that can produce renal failure. Determination of the etiology is extremely important, because the treatment will depend on the underlying cause.

The normal physiologic changes of pregnancy add a layer of complexity to evaluating renal failure in the parturient compared with the nonpregnant patient. During pregnancy, kidneys can normally undergo a 30% increase in size, and hydronephrosis may cause an even further enlargement. The glomerular filtration rate (GFR) will increase to 30% to 50% more than in nonpregnant women, primarily owing to a reduced average oncotic pressure and an increase in ultrafiltration, and renal plasma flow will initially increase beyond and then decrease below the GFR, leading to increased filtration toward the end of pregnancy.[6] The normally occurring changes in renal physiology during pregnancy lead to increased an intravascular volume owing to hormonal changes, a normal increase in protein excretion of up to 300 mg/24 h, an increase in creatinine clearance to 120 to 160 mL/min, and a decrease in serum creatinine to 0.4 to 0.7 mg/dL.[1,7]

Because the increased GFR and hemodilution from increasing intravascular volume during pregnancy causes an expected decrease in serum creatinine, there is an intrinsic inaccuracy in applying commonly used measures to evaluate renal disease in the case of pregnancy. The Modification of Diet in Renal Disease formula that is frequently used to estimate GFR in patients with chronic kidney disease underestimates the GFR when the GFR is greater than 60 mL/min/m,[2] and the Cockcroft–Gault formula for estimating GFR is weight based, and tends to overestimate GFR in the pregnant patient owing to increased body weight not being from increased muscle mass.[8] For these reasons, the gold standard for estimating GFR in the pregnant patient is 24-hour urine collection for creatinine clearance. It is also useful to establish whether a decrease in the GFR is secondary to renal vasoconstriction or systemic hypoperfusion with intact tubular function or established ARF. A fractional excretion of filtered sodium (FE_{Na} = [(urine sodium × plasma creatinine)/(plasma sodium × urine creatinine)]) of less then 1% is indicative of preserved tubular sodium reabsorbtion and intact tubular function.

Although a renal biopsy may be useful in nonpregnant patients, it tends to be less useful in the evaluation of pregnant patients owing to there being a higher chance of already knowing the underlying etiology. The major role of biopsy is for the identification of renal failure not owing to preeclampsia, to find a therapy other than delivery.[2]

ETIOLOGY

The etiology of renal failure is best classified as prerenal (owing to decreased renal perfusion), intrarenal (owing to specific effects on the renal parenchyma), or postrenal (usually owing to obstruction). Prerenal causes of acute failure (**Box 1**) are usually owing to hypovolemia from obstetric hemorrhage (owing to abortion, placenta previa, placental abruption, uterine rupture or postpartum hemorrhage), but may also occur owing to severe cases of hyperemesis gravidarum, leading to prerenal ischemia from decreased renal perfusion, and from amniotic fluid embolism leading to disseminated intravascular coagulation, cardiac dysfunction, and hemorrhage causing intravascular volume depletion and reduced renal perfusion.[2] When renal ischemia is prolonged and persistent, acute tubular necrosis (ATN) develops owing to necrosis or apoptosis of the most active tubular cells. The combination of parenchymal edema and the sloughing of necrotic tubular epithelium into the tubule obstructs the tubular lumen, leading to resultant decreased GFR and granular casts in the urinary sediment.[5]

Sepsis can lead to hypotension and decreased renal perfusion, with resultant prerenal ischemia, and potentially to ATN. The most common causes are pyelonephritis, chorioamnionitis, and pneumonia, and there is an increased risk of renal failure owing to pyelonephritis, even independent of sepsis. Pyelonephritis itself is associated with a greater risk of systemic inflammation and sepsis owing to ureteral dilation, bladder wall flaccidity, and increased sensitivity to bacterial endotoxin induced tissue damage.[2] A septic state may be more difficult to diagnose in the pregnant patient owing to the normal increase in white blood cell count during pregnancy, increased temperature with neuraxial labor analgesia, and the increased heart rate and respiration rate that occur during labor. The most commonly encountered pathogens are endotoxin-producing Gram-negative rods, and in many cases the infection is polymicrobial such as with *Escherichia coli*, enterococci, *Klebsiella*, *Staphylococcus aureus*, and β-hemolytic streptococci.[9]

Intrarenal causes of renal failure in pregnancy are varied as listed in **Box 2**. Preeclampsia is a severe systemic disease of pregnancy that is a major cause of maternal morbidity and mortality. Mild preeclampsia has historically referred to a condition in which there is persistent systolic blood pressure of greater than 140 mm Hg and/or a diastolic blood pressure of greater than 90 mm Hg, and proteinuria of greater than 300 mg/24 h after 20 weeks gestation, although the American College of Obstetricians and Gynecologists has recently stated that proteinuria is no longer necessary for the diagnosis of preeclampsia. Severe hypertension with a systolic blood pressure greater than 160 mm Hg and/or a diastolic blood pressure of greater than 110 mm Hg, proteinuria of greater than 5 g/24 h and systemic involvement such as the hemolysis, elevated liver enzymes, and low platelet count (HELLP) syndrome, renal failure, neurologic symptoms, and acute pulmonary edema are criteria for the severity of disease.[10]

Box 1
Prerenal causes of renal failure in pregnancy
Hemorrhage
Hyperemesis gravidarum
Sepsis
Amniotic fluid embolism

Box 2
Intrarenal causes of renal failure in pregnancy

Preexisting renal disease

Ischemia

Preeclampsia and hemolysis, elevated liver enzymes, and low platelet count (HELLP) syndrome

Thrombotic microangiopathies

Acute fatty liver of pregnancy

- About 40% of ARF in pregnancy is owing to severe preeclampsia and HELLP, and up to 20% of women with severe preeclampsia develop HELLP. ARF occurs in about 1% of women with severe preeclampsia and 3% to 15% of women with HELLP, with renal failure usually occurring antepartum or early postpartum.[11]
- Patients are predisposed to ARF through volume depletion, vasoconstriction, and inflammatory and coagulation cascades activation. The pathognomonic histologic lesion is glomeruloendotheliosis, with decreased glomerular size, increased cytoplasmic volume, decreased capillary lumen diameter, and sometimes complete obstruction, and the primary pathologic process is ATN, with the most severe cases at risk for renal cortical necrosis.[2]
- Piccoli and colleagues[12] showed that in the presence of proteinuria and hypertension, abnormal uterine and umbilical Doppler flow velocities indicate a diagnosis of preeclampsia, whereas normal flow velocities indicate a diagnosis of chronic kidney disease.

Acute fatty liver of pregnancy (AFLP) is a condition with rapidly progressive hepatic failure in late gestation and occurs with nausea, vomiting, malaise, and mental status changes. Laboratory abnormalities include hyperbilirubinemia, elevated transaminases, elevated ammonia levels, and hypoglycemia.[2] It has an incidence of 1 in 7000 to 1 in 20,000 pregnancies, has a maternal mortality of 0% to 12.5%, and fetal and perinatal mortality of 6.6% to 15%. Coagulopathy is seen with hyperfibrinogenemia, prolonged prothrombin time, depressed antithrombin III levels and thrombocytopenia. There is a coexisting ARF in 20% to 100% of cases, and it generally presents as a nonoliguric ARF, although oliguria can occur with hemorrhage-induced hypovolemia. Renal biopsy shows mild glomerular hypercellularity with thick narrow capillary loops and tubular free fatty acid oxidation. Proteinuria and peripheral edema are common owing to coexisting preeclampsia, which can occur in up to 50% of women with AFLP. They share similar pathophysiology and clinical symptoms, and may in fact be in the same spectrum of illness.[11]

Thrombotic thrombocytopenic purpura (TTP) and hemolytic uremic syndrome (HUS) are thrombotic microangiopathies in which thrombi of fibrin and/or platelets occur in the organ microvasculature, primarily the brain and kidney. Histologic findings in the kidney show endothelial cell swelling, subendothelial protein deposits, and double contouring of the basement membrane. Whereas HUS mainly affects the kidney, TTP usually presents as severe thrombocytopenia with neurologic disturbances, but the 2 disease processes tend to overlap in their presentation.[13]

- Laboratory testing checks for signs of microangiopathic hemolytic anemia, thrombocytopenia, red cell fragmentation on peripheral smear, elevated lactate dehydrogenase, and indirect hyperbilirubinemia.[9]

- The incidence is 1 in 25,000 births, and median gestational age at onset is 23 weeks, which is usually earlier than preeclampsia, although they can occur at anytime during pregnancy or postpartum. These conditions share similarities with and may be difficult to differentiate from severe preeclampsia, and are often diagnosed post partum after an initial diagnosis of severe preeclampsia.[2]
- TTP is usually caused by an acquired or an inherent deficiency of the von Willebrand factor cleaving metalloproteinase ADAMTS13, whereas HUS tends to be caused by dysregulation of C3 convertase with uncontrolled activation of complement system leading to endothelial damage in the kidney.[13]
- Although ADAMTS13 deficiency is associated with TTP in the nonpregnant patient, it is not well-studied in TTP associated with pregnancy. It is know, however, that levels of ADAMTS13 decrease from 94% in first trimester to 64% in second and third trimesters in normal pregnancy, and may decrease to as low as 5% in pregnancy-associated TTP.[11]
- The absence of coagulation abnormalities such as elevated antithrombin, elevated D-dimer, and high fibrinogen, levels are suggestive of TTP rather than preeclampsia, but levels of ADAMTS13 may be normal in TTP and low in HELLP.

Postrenal causes of renal failure in pregnancy are obstruction, surgical injury or drug effect (**Box 3**). Although urinary stasis and compression of the urinary system are common during pregnancy, renal failure owing to obstruction is a relatively rare entity, although it may occur as the uterus compresses the genitourinary system, particularly with polyhydramnios, multiple gestation, and uterine fibroids.[1,2] Although quite rare, ureteral injury such as by ligation or transection may occur during caesarean section. There is the potential for postoperative uremia when this injury leads to a total interruption of the urinary flow, with anuria being the only immediate sign of imminent uremia.[14] Drugs commonly used in pregnancy such as sulfonamides and acyclovir may also lead to postrenal renal failure.[1]

TREATMENT

Treatment success of renal failure in pregnancy primarily depends on providing supportive measures, quick and accurate assessment and correction of the underlying etiology, and prevention of further damage and deterioration. As in the nonpregnant patient, fluid management is the most important initial therapy for ARF, with the goal of restoring and maintaining urine output and renal perfusion to reverse preischemic changes and to limit further damage, even after tubular necrosis has occurred.[1,2]

- It has been suggested that the use of lactated Ringer's solution and Plasmalyte is associated with less renal injury than normal saline because higher concentrations chloride can lead to vasoconstriction and ischemia.[1]
- Additional important steps include the removal and avoidance of nephrotoxins, adjustment of medication dosing for renal clearance (particularly magnesium),

Box 3
Postrenal causes of renal failure in pregnancy
Obstruction
Surgical injury
Drugs

and the prevention and treatment of infection because sepsis is the most common cause of mortality of in ARF.[2]

- Overt blood loss should be replaced early because hemorrhage near term may be hard to detect, and early and appropriate management can prevent or limit irreversible change.[2,15]
- For some etiologies like preeclampsia and AFLP, all measures are supportive because delivery is the only definitive therapy.

PHARMACOLOGIC TREATMENT OPTIONS

In general, pharmacologic therapy is considered second line for ARF, and the use of pharmacologic therapy to maintain perfusion and urinary output has not been associated with improved outcomes. Although various pharmacotherapies have been suggested to increase renal blood flow and maintain urinary output, there is little evidence that they provide any benefit. The use of dopamine infusion, loop diuretics, systemic vasodilator atrial natriuretic peptide, fenoldopam, and N-acetylcysteine for the maintenance of urinary output have been studied, and have not shown any benefit in the treatment of ARF.[1,2] Although diuretic use leads to decreased intravascular volume, which may inhibit labor and decrease placental perfusion, thiazide diuretics may be indicated for severe intractable preeclampsia or pulmonary edema. Although serum albumin levels are often found to be low and infusions have been shown to increase both serum albumin and colloid osmotic pressures, it does not stabilize renal function and was associated with higher fetal mortality.[16] Although mannitol should theoretically be beneficial in preventing ARF in high-risk patients, no trials have been done in pregnant women to assess the efficacy.[5]

In the case of renal failure occurring secondary to a state of sepsis and shock, important tenets of therapy include early antibiotic administration to maintain source control, and broad empiric coverage with vancomycin and meropenem is commonly employed until the determination can be made for a more specific antibiotic therapy.[9] When treating septic abortion or chorioamnionitis, evacuation of the uterine contents is necessary for effective treatment because antibiotic penetration of the uterine cavity is suboptimal.[2]

The various complications of renal failure and the underlying etiologies should be treated pharmacologically when appropriate.

- Hypertension is commonly treated with methyldopa and labetalol, as well as dihydropyridine calcium channel blockers; other commonly used antihypertensives are contraindicated in pregnancy. Hyperkalemia can be treated with insulin, glucose, and ion exchange resin.[17]
- The management of potassium and phosphate imbalances is similar to that of the nonpregnant patient.[1]

Because renal failure occurring during pregnancy is not one specific entity, but rather a result of a variety of processes, pharmacotherapy must be tailored to the underlying etiology. Women experiencing hyperemesis gravidarum should receive thiamine supplementation, and a variety of medications can be used to control nausea, including dopamine antagonists, phenothiazines, histamine receptor blockers, and corticosteroids.[18]

When preeclampsia is the underlying etiology leading to renal failure, treatment is primarily supportive and the only definitive therapy is delivery.

- Corticosteroids have been suggested as a possible pharmacotherapy, but trials have shown no benefit with regard to duration of hospitalization, recovery speed, or development of complications.[17]

- Despite the existence of peripheral edema, decreasing intravascular volume is not recommended and diuretics may inhibit labor and decrease placental perfusion, although the use of thiazide diuretics may be indicated for severe intractable preeclampsia or pulmonary edema. Lowering uric acid with probenecid has no effect on hypertension in preeclampsia, and allopurinol therapy has no effect on pregnancy outcome.[16]
- Magnesium sulfate delivered intravenously is the most important pharmacotherapy for the prevention of progression to seizures. Although tending to be rare, side effects can be quite severe, including loss of patellar reflexes, respiratory depression, and cardiac dysfunction, and extra care should be taken to monitor magnesium levels and urine output in the patient with existing renal failure because magnesium excretion may be decreased.[11,19]
- Lorazepam and phenytoin may be used for refractory seizures not responsive to magnesium therapy.[16]

For TTP and HUS, steroids are recommended as the initial immunosuppressive therapy in the cases of a suspected ADAMTS-13 deficiency. The use of cyclosporine, rituximab, and vincristine has been reported in more severe cases, and the use of heparin anticoagulation is potentially harmful.[2,17] Fresh frozen plasma can be given for the correction of ADAMTS-13 deficiency.[17]

When AFLP is the underlying etiology, therapies consist of stabilizing maternal glucose with dextrose, correction of anemia and coagulopathy with blood transfusion, fresh frozen plasma, and cryoprecipitate, and treatment of hepatic encephalopathy with a low protein diet and oral lactulose.[11,17] As with preeclampsia, treatment is mainly supportive, and delivery is the definitive therapy.

NONPHARMACOLOGIC TREATMENT OPTIONS

Renal failure can progress to the point of requiring dialysis to prevent maternal morbidity and mortality, and allow for progression of pregnancy to a point where delivery is feasible. It is a purely supportive measure, and there is no evidence that it shortens the course of ARF.[5] Both peritoneal dialysis and hemodialysis have been used successfully to treat renal failure occurring during pregnancy.[20] Although there are no studies to determine the optimal mode of dialysis in the pregnant patient, intermittent hemodialysis is the most commonly chosen modality, although continuous hemofiltration has come into use more recently, because it allows for control of volume and solute loads, and to prevent the hemodynamic fluctuations that occur with intermittent dialysis.[2,17] Dialysis should be undertaken early because urea, creatinine, and other metabolites that accumulate can cross the placenta, and fetal survival and gestational age are improved with a lower serum blood urea nitrogen and creatinine.[15,20] Indications for initiating dialysis include uremic symptoms, volume overload, and metabolic acidosis and hyperkalemia unresponsive to medical therapy, although other recommended parameters are serum creatinine of 3.5 to 5.0 mg/dL or GFR decreasing to less than 20 mL/min (**Box 4**).[17,20] The placement of a peritoneal dialysis catheter is technically feasible in pregnancy, and the peritoneal membrane has been shown to maintain clearance and ultrafiltration capabilities. There are a number of advantages with peritoneal dialysis, including minimizing fluid and electrolyte shifts, reduction of hypotension, better management of hypertension, and the ability to administer insulin and magnesium as needed.

- Although plasmapheresis is likely not helpful for most causes of ARF, it is used therapeutically for thrombotic microangiopathies by clearing large thrombogenic

> **Box 4**
> **Indications for dialysis for renal failure in pregnancy**
>
> Symptomatic uremia (encephalopathy, pericarditis, neuropathy)
>
> Volume overload
>
> Hyperkalemia
>
> Metabolic acidosis
>
> Serum creatinine 3.5 to 5.0 mg/dL
>
> Glomerular filtration rate of <20 mL/min

multimers or autoantibodies,[1] and plasma infusion and plasma exchange are used to treat atypical HUS.[17]

- No trials have been done studying plasma exchange for preeclampsia/HELLP, but it seems to be an option with low risk during pregnancy and may be promising for otherwise refractory preeclampsia.[11,16]
- There is no strong evidence for plasma exchange to treat AFLP, but the use of molecular adsorbent recirculating systems may present a new mode of therapy.[11]

SURGICAL TREATMENT OPTIONS

When renal failure occurs as a result of obstruction, treatment includes procedures to relieve the obstruction such as cystoscopy, stents, and percutaneous nephrostomy.[1] In the case of severe preeclampsia, uterine curettage immediately after delivery can accelerate recovery.[16] Definitive surgical therapy after the failure of all other therapies is eventual renal transplantation.

EVALUATION OF OUTCOME AND LONG-TERM RECOMMENDATIONS

Patient outcome depends mainly on the underlying cause, the degree of severity of the renal failure, and associated complications. Mortality rates range from 20% to 80%, and between 5% and 30% of those requiring dialysis require it long term.[5] Recovery after ATN is largely depends on how much damage has occurred and how much of the nephron remains unaffected, as well as the maintenance of urine output indicates a milder injury.[1]

ARF occurs in in about 3% of severe HELLP cases, typically with ATN, and tends to develop when severe complications are present, such as placental abruption, disseminated intravascular coagulation, sepsis, postpartum bleeding, or fetal death. The likelihood of renal failure increases with severity of HELLP. Although maternal mortality in HELLP is about 1% and up to 13% with coexisting renal failure, perinatal mortality in HELLP ranges from 7% to 20% and up to 26% with coexisting renal failure.[11] Among pregnancy-related diseases, HELLP syndrome associated with postpartum hemorrhage has the highest risk of ARF in the complicated postpartum setting.[21]

- Although as many as 30% to 50% of those who develop renal failure with HELLP will require dialysis on a temporary basis, renal function generally improves after delivery. Despite this improvement, more than 50% of women with preeclampsia will develop hypertension later in life, and the relative risk of subsequent ischemic heart disease, stroke, and cardiovascular mortality is more than doubled. The risk of progression to end-stage renal disease may be increased by almost 5-fold.[11]

- Although it is rare for previously healthy preeclampsia patients to required long-term dialysis, patients with preexisting hypertension or renal disease are significantly more likely to require long-term dialysis.[2]
- Complications occurring in the fetus and neonate owing to severe preeclampsia include fetal growth restriction (10%–25%), hypoxia-induced neurologic damage (<1%), and perinatal death (1.2%). Discontinuance of pregnancy is recommended before 24 weeks gestation for cases of severe preeclampsia and HELLP, because there is no evidence of fetal survival benefit and there is an increased risk of severe maternal complications. Expectant management may be undertaken between 24 and 32 weeks gestation. For pregnancies greater than 32 weeks, delivery is the recommended treatment. Worsening maternal condition, eclampsia, and fetal compromise are indications for delivery, regardless of gestational age.[17]

Up to two-thirds of cases of thrombotic microangiopathies will have renal involvement, although HUS is typically associated with severe ARF and the frequent need for dialysis, and TTP is usually associated with only mild renal insufficiency.[1,17]

- Perinatal mortality is as high as 30% to 80%, and although maternal mortality has decreased to 10% to 20%, 76% of patients will progress to end-stage kidney disease, and the need for chronic dialysis or renal transplant is not uncommon.[11,17]
- Pregnancy outcomes include fetal growth restriction, fetal distress, intrauterine demise, and recurrence with future pregnancy.[2]
- Plasma exchange has been found to decrease mortality from 90% to 10% in TTP, and is standard of care for pregnancy associated TTP.[11]
- Although therapy is primarily supportive and delivery does not influence disease remission, it should be induced for serious illness.[17]

About 60% of patients with AFLP will develop ARF, and although most women with AFLP will have full recovery of liver and kidney function after delivery, there is a maternal and perinatal mortality of 10% to 20%.[1,17] Because renal recovery tends to be complete after delivery, dialysis is rarely needed, although early diagnosis and immediate delivery are essential to avoid progression to renal failure.[11,17] For renal failure owing to obstruction, there is excellent prognosis for general recovery and restoration of renal function after relief of the obstruction, and the need for dialysis is rare.[2]

Hladunewich and colleagues[22] found that intensive hemodialysis leads to a higher proportion of live infants, greater median gestational age and birth weight, and reduced maternal and neonatal complications. They speculate that their findings indicate that intensified dialysis dose provides a healthy maternal environment for normal placental development, allowing for normal fetal growth and decreased pregnancy complications. A daily dialysis program (>20 hours per week) should be established to improve uremia, minimize hemodialysis-induced hemodynamic fluctuations, and avoid excessive fluid removal, because these conditions can lead to premature labor, polyhydramnios, hemodynamic compromise, uteroplacental perfusion, and placental oxidative stress.[15,17] Dialysis schedules should aim for a predialysis urea of 30 to 50 mg/dL. Consideration should be given to polyhydramnios being a complication of high maternal urea, leading to high urea and solute diuresis by the fetus, which can contribute to premature labor.

SUMMARY

Renal failure in pregnancy is a rare but severe complication that can have significant long-term effects on both the mother and the fetus. Evaluation of the pregnant patient must take into consideration the normal physiologic changes of pregnancy that increase the complexity of diagnosing renal failure. The etiology of renal failure in the pregnant patient is best divided into prerenal, intrarenal, and postrenal causes, with the focus of treatment based on the underlying cause. Supportive measures such as fluid resuscitation are the basis of treatment for renal failure in pregnancy, with delivery usually being the ultimate goal. When other measures fail dialysis may be required, with the goal of prolonging pregnancy until delivery becomes feasible, and providing an environment suitable for fetal growth.

REFERENCES

1. Van Hook JW. Acute kidney injury during pregnancy. Clin Obstet Gynecol 2014; 57(4):851–61.
2. Gammill HS, Jeyabalan A. Acute renal failure in pregnancy. Crit Care Med 2005; 33(10 Suppl):S372–84.
3. Thadhani R, Pascual M, Bonventre JV. Acute renal failure. N Engl J Med 1996; 334(22):1448–60.
4. Bellomo R, Ronco C, Kellum JA, et al. Acute renal failure - definition, outcome measures, animal models, fluid therapy and information technology needs: the Second International Consensus Conference of the Acute Dialysis Quality Initiative (ADQI) Group. Crit Care 2004;8(4):R204–12.
5. Mantel GD. Care of the critically ill parturient: oliguria and renal failure. Best Pract Res Clin Obstet Gynaecol 2001;15(4):563–81.
6. Hussein W, Lafayette RA. Renal function in normal and disordered pregnancy. Curr Opin Nephrol Hypertens 2014;23(1):46–53.
7. Munnur U, Bandi V, Guntupalli KK. Management principles of the critically ill obstetric patient. Clin Chest Med 2011;32(1):53–60, viii.
8. Maynard SE, Thadhani R. Pregnancy and the kidney. J Am Soc Nephrol 2009; 20(1):14–22. Available at: http://jasn.asnjournals.org/content/20/1/14.long.
9. Galvagno SM Jr, Camann W. Sepsis and acute renal failure in pregnancy. Anesth Analg 2009;108(2):572–5.
10. Lambert G, Brichant JF, Hartstein G, et al. Preeclampsia: an update. Acta Anaesthesiol Belg 2014;65(4):137–49.
11. Ganesan C, Maynard SE. Acute kidney injury in pregnancy: the thrombotic microangiopathies. J Nephrol 2011;24(5):554–63.
12. Piccoli GB, Gaglioti P, Attini R, et al. Pre-eclampsia or chronic kidney disease? the flow hypothesis. Nephrol Dial Transplant 2013;28(5):1199–206.
13. Fakhouri F, Vercel C, Frémeaux-Bacchi V. Obstetric nephrology: AKI and thrombotic microangiopathies in pregnancy. Clin J Am Soc Nephrol 2012;7(12): 2100–6.
14. Jha S, Coomarasamy A, Chan K. Ureteric injury in obstetric and gynaecological surgery. The Obstetrician & Gynaecologist 2004;6:203–8.
15. Podymow T, August P, Akbari A. Management of renal disease in pregnancy. Obstet Gynecol Clin North Am 2010;37(2):195–210.
16. Müller-Deile J, Schiffer M. Preeclampsia from a renal point of view: Insides into disease models, biomarkers and therapy. World J Nephrol 2014;3(4):169–81.
17. Machado S, Figueiredo N, Borges A, et al. Acute kidney injury in pregnancy: a clinical challenge. J Nephrol 2012;25(1):19–30.

18. Wegrzyniak LJ, Repke JT, Ural SH. Treatment of hyperemesis gravidarum. Rev Obstet Gynecol 2012;5(2):78–84.

19. Smith JM, Lowe RF, Fullerton J, et al. An integrative review of the side effects related to the use of magnesium sulfate for pre-eclampsia and eclampsia management. BMC Pregnancy Childbirth 2013;13:34.

20. Krane N. Peritoneal dialysis and hemodialysis in pregnancy. Hemodial Int 2001;5: 97–101.

21. Jonard M, Ducloy-Bouthors AS, Boyle E, et al. Postpartum acute renal failure: a multicenter study of risk factors in patients admitted to ICU. Ann Intensive Care 2014;4:36.

22. Hladunewich MA, Hou S, Odutayo A, et al. Intensive hemodialysis associates with improved pregnancy outcomes: a Canadian and United States cohort comparison. J Am Soc Nephrol 2014;25(5):1103–9.

Respiratory Failure and Mechanical Ventilation in the Pregnant Patient

David Schwaiberger, MD[a],*, Marcin Karcz, MD, MSc[b],
Mario Menk, MD[a], Peter J. Papadakos, MD[c],
Susan E. Dantoni, MD[d,e]

KEYWORDS

- Respiratory failure • Pregnancy • ARDS • Mechanical ventilation
- Noninvasive ventilation

KEY POINTS

- Several physiologic and anatomic changes in pregnancy promote the incidence of respiratory failure. The fetus needs a maternal Pao_2 greater than 70 mm Hg for sufficient oxygenation.
- Common causes of respiratory failure in pregnancy are pneumonia, different kinds of pulmonary edema, exacerbation of asthma, aspiration, pulmonary embolism, amniotic fluid syndrome, and pneumothorax.
- Acute respiratory distress syndrome is a severe complication of all mentioned respiratory diseases and may lead to support with extracorporeal membrane oxygenation.
- Intubation failure is frequent in pregnant patients. Mechanical ventilation should be applied as in nonpregnant patients. Higher peak pressure and positive end expiratory pressure may lead to normal transpulmonary pressure.
- Noninvasive ventilation is an option in alert patients in the hands of a skilled therapist.

Potential Conflict of Interest: All authors have nothing to report.
[a] Department of Anesthesiology and Intensive Care Medicine, Charité - University Medicine Berlin, Campus Charité Mitte and Campus Virchow-Klinikum, Augustenburger Platz 1, Berlin 13353, Germany; [b] Department of Anesthesiology, University of Rochester School of Medicine, 601 Elmwood Avenue, Rochester, NY 14642, USA; [c] Department of Anesthesiology, University of Rochester School of Medicine, University of Rochester Medical Center, Box 604, Rochester, NY 14642, USA; [d] Bellevue Women's Center/Ellis Hospital, Schenectady, New York, USA; [e] Department OB/GYN, Albany Medical College, 47 New Scotland Ave, Albany, NY 12208, USA
* Corresponding author.
E-mail address: david.schwaiberger@charite.de

Crit Care Clin 32 (2016) 85–95
http://dx.doi.org/10.1016/j.ccc.2015.08.001
0749-0704/16/$ – see front matter © 2016 Elsevier Inc. All rights reserved.

INTRODUCTION

Acute respiratory failure with need of ventilator support is rare in pregnant patients. Fewer than 2% of women in the peripartal period need treatment in the intensive care unit (ICU). The main diseases that lead to ICU admission in nondeveloping countries are hypertensive diseases, hemorrhage, and sepsis.[1,2] Respiratory failure is a common complication of these and other diseases in the obstetric or postpartum patient; therefore, respiratory failure is one of the main indications for ICU admission.

PHYSIOLOGIC CHANGES OF RESPIRATORY SYSTEM IN PREGNANCY

Pregnancy leads to anatomic and physiologic changes of lung and the respiratory system that can promote respiratory failure.

Changes regarding the respiratory system are[3] as follows:

- Edema and hyperemia of the upper airways
- Reduced tonus of the lower esophagus sphincter
- Increased respiratory drive with greater tidal volume leading to increased minute ventilation due to elevated levels of progesterone
- Decreased functional residual capacity (FRC)
- Elevated diaphragm due to the enlarging uterus (up to 5 cm)
- Decreased compliance of the ventilatory system (reduction of chest wall compliance, lung compliance is unaltered)
- Increased O_2 consumption and CO_2 production due to the demands of the fetus
- Respiratory alkalosis with a decrease of bicarbonate

DETERMINANTS OF OXYGEN DELIVERY AND HYPOXEMIA IN THE FETUS

The oxygen delivery to the fetus is determined by the following:

- Uterine blood flow
- Maternal arterial oxygen content
- Concentration of maternal hemoglobin
- The hemoglobin–oxygen-dissociation curve of mother and the fetus.[4]

The adequate oxygen content for the fetus is maintained by a left shift of the oxygen-dissociation curve of fetal hemoglobin; the umbilical venous blood returning to the fetus has a Pao_2 of only 25 to 30 mm Hg.[5]

Maternal hypoxia results in fetoplacental vasoconstriction, which reduces placental blood flow and fetal oxygen transfer.[6] Placental vasoconstriction also can be provoked by endogenous or exogenous catecholamines, alkalosis, hypotension, and contractions.[7]

A theoretic model based on animal studies showed that a maternal O_2 saturation of 95% to 88% resulted in a fetal saturation of 70% to 55%.[8] However, maternal hypoxemia with an inhalation of 10% O_2 for 10 minutes showed no adverse effect in fetal monitoring.[9]

Hypocapnia also results in decrease of uterine blood flow,[10] whereas mild hypercapnia showed no effect on uterine blood flow, and a higher $Paco_2$ is associated with a better APGAR score.[11]

CAUSES OF RESPIRATORY FAILURE IN PREGNANCY
Pneumonia

Pneumonia in pregnancy is still the third leading cause of indirect obstetric maternal death.[12,13] In most cases, community-acquired pneumonia and viral pneumonia are the main admission diagnoses in this group to hospital or ICU.

The most frequent pathogens are *Streptococcus pneumoniae, Haemophilus influenzae*, and atypical pathogens like *Mycoplasma pneumoniae, Legionella pneumoniae, Chlamydia pneumoniae*, varicella, and influenza A.[14]

Maternal asthma, history of other pulmonary diseases, and anemia with a hemoglobin level of 10 g/dL or lower are associated with pneumonia.[15]

Clinical symptoms are as follows:

- Dyspnea
- Fever
- Cough productive sputum
- Pleural chest pain
- Nausea
- Headache
- Myalgia
- Changes in mental status

Because of the unspecific symptoms, pneumonia in pregnancy is often misdiagnosed and the adequate therapy is delayed.[16]

If there is a clinical suspicion, the diagnosis should be verified by chest radiograph and sputum cultures should be used to verify the pathogen. In laboratory tests, a leukocytosis with a left shift is typical. In urine tests, antigens of *S pneumoniae* and *L pneumoniae* can be detected.

The first choice of treatment is antibiotic therapy with a macrolide, such as azithromycin. If necessary, this should be amended by a beta-lactam against pneumococci, especially if the hospital's local resistance against macrolides is higher than 25%. Tetracyclines should be avoided in pregnancy. If gram-negative germs such as *Pseudomonas aeruginosa* are suspected, an aminoglycoside should be added.

Pregnant patients with high risk or strong suspicion of influenza A should be treated with oseltamivir starting in the first 48 hours of disease according to the Centers for Disease Control and Prevention guidelines.[17] Most severe cases are not vaccinated, but antiviral treatment should be applied regardless of test results or vaccination status.[18]

Varicella pneumonia also plays an important role in pneumonia in pregnancy due to decreased cell-mediated immunity in the last trimenon[19]; thus, women of childbearing age should be vaccinated as soon as possible.

In some cases, mechanical ventilation or noninvasive ventilation will be necessary.

Exacerbation of Asthma

Up to 8% of pregnant women suffer from asthma.[20] One-third of these patients have 1 or more exacerbations of asthma during pregnancy.[21]

Pregnant women with asthma have a higher risk of the following:

- Low birth weight
- Small gestational age
- Preterm birth
- Congenital malformations
- Preeclampsia
- Neonatal hospitalization
- Neonatal death

The most complications occur because of medication incompliance. It should be emphasized that corticoid medication is not absolutely contraindicated in pregnancy, and uncontrolled asthma does more harm to the fetus than asthma medication.

Inhaled corticoids should be preferred, but, systemically, corticoids should be administrated if necessary. Patient education is necessary and essential to prevent exacerbation of chronic asthma.

Besides corticoid medication, beta-agonists can be used, but they inhibit labor.

Close monitoring of mother and fetus is necessary recognize and prevent severe asthma.

Often asthma coexists with gastroesophageal reflux disease, which should be treated with proton-pump inhibitors such as omeprazole.[22]

Pulmonary Edema

Pulmonary edema in pregnancy can occur due to cardiac dysfunction or to the use of tocolytic agents or corticoid medication, respectively. Additionally, pulmonary edema is a rare complication of preeclampsia.[23]

Reduced vascular tonus, decrease of plasma proteins, and increase of blood volume predispose pregnant women for pulmonary edema.[24]

The tocolytic pulmonary edema arises in the first 24 hours after administration of beta-2-agonists, such as terbutaline, albuterol, or ritodrine. In rare cases, magnesium sulfate or calcium channel blockers can lead to a pulmonary edema.

Cardiac dysfunction can be a result of preexisting or new heart diseases, such as valvular dysfunction, cardiomyopathies, or myocardial dysfunction.

The pathogenesis of pulmonary edema in preeclampsia is not yet clear, but it seems to be multifactorial. Fluid overload is the main reason in most kinds of pulmonary edema, but cardiac dysfunction and increased capillary permeability are of importance.

Exploration of pulmonary edema should be made by echocardiography to discriminate between cardiac and noncardiac causes.

Treatment of pulmonary edema, besides supplementation of oxygen, could be administration of diuretics and inotrope agents in cardiac failure. Of course, in tocolytic pulmonary edema, the infusion of beta-2-agonists should be stopped and other tocolytics should be used. Noninvasive ventilation and continuous positive airway pressure are helpful in treating patients with pulmonary edema.

Aspiration

The risk of aspiration rises in pregnancy due to increase of abdominal pressure, relaxation of the lower esophagus sphincter, and delayed gastric emptying. Aspiration can lead to acute bronchospasm, airway obstruction, and finally, in most cases, to a chemical pneumonitis (Mendelson syndrome) or an aspiration pneumonia.

In contrast to pneumonia, chemical pneumonitis has a rapid onset with productive cough (gastric content), diffuse crackles in auscultation, and basal infiltrates in the chest radiograph. Fever is low grade.

A few minutes after aspiration, atelectasis, hemorrhage, and pulmonary edema occur, and within hours, the alveolar space is filled with leukocytes and fibrin. This leads to formation of hyaline membranes. Chemical pneumonitis has 3 potential outcomes: rapid recovery, an acute respiratory distress syndrome (ARDS)-like picture, or a bacterial superinfection, the aspiration pneumonia.[25]

Aspiration pneumonia is mostly caused by anaerobic germs, but a wide spectrum of microorganisms provoking aspiration pneumonia is known. This depends on the patient's setting, especially the length of hospital stay and the hospital-specific problematic germs. The first step of anti-infective treatment is penicillin, such as amoxicillin or ampicillin.

Besides ventilator support, treatment in the ICU includes bronchoscopy with suctioning of the aspirated material, particularly if there is airway obstruction.

Pulmonary Embolism

In pregnancy, the risk for pulmonary embolism (PE) events rises 5 to 6 times[26] and is the main reason for cardiopulmonary resuscitation (CPR) in this period. The highest risk is in the postpartum period.[27]

Several factors promote PE in pregnancy:

- Changes of clotting factors with decrease of Protein S and increase of procoagulatory factors (I, II, VII, VIII, IX, and X) promote hypercoagulability
- Pressure by the uterus on the vena cava inferior results in venous stasis
- Endothelial injury during pregnancy (eg, delivery)[28]

The clinical symptoms are various, as in nonpregnant patients. In most cases, dyspnea, tachycardia, and chest pain emerge. Hypotension and shock are symptoms if right heart failure appears.

D-Dimer is not reliable in pregnancy.[29]

The diagnosis should be confirmed with computed tomography with pulmonary angiography and echocardiography to evaluate the right ventricular function.

The cornerstone in therapy of PE besides cardiopulmonary stabilization is an effective anticoagulation with low-molecular-weight heparin (LMWH) for at least 3 months. Anti-Xa level should be checked frequently. LMWH does not cross the placenta.

Coumarins, such as warfarin, should not be used in pregnancy because they are teratogen and can cause fetal bleeding.[30]

In severe life-threating cases, thrombolysis is an option, but the risk of maternal bleeding (8%) or fetal loss (6%) is high.[31]

Air Embolism

Venous air embolism occurs if the pressure of the right heart is lower than the pressure on the open vessel. This is most common in sectio caesarea, but also can develop in central line placement, abortions, or other obstetric procedures.[32]

Symptoms are similar to PE; respiratory and circulatory supportive treatment is needed. In severe cases, hyperbaric oxygen therapy could be necessary.[33]

Pneumothorax in Trauma

Domestic violence and motor vehicle accidents are the predominant causes of trauma in pregnancy. Trauma is the leading cause of maternal death in the United States.[34] Thoracic trauma with flail chest could result in pneumothorax with sudden dyspnea, loss of ventilation sounds in auscultation, and hypotension, if a tension pneumothorax emerges.

Treatment of pneumothorax is to drain the pleura with a chest tube. Because of the elevated diaphragm in pregnancy, it is recommended to insert the chest tube 1 to 2 intercostal spaces above the known landmark of the fifth intercostal space to avoid abdominal placement.[35] After insertion, the position of the chest tube should be verified by chest radiograph.

Amniotic Fluid Embolism

Amniotic fluid embolism (AFE) is a rare, but catastrophic event in the intrapartum or early postpartum period, with a maternal mortality of 11% to 86%.[36]

During delivery, amniotic fluid is entering the circulation through endocervical veins, and provokes the following:

- Cardiogenic shock with acute pulmonary hypertension and left ventricular failure as a result of vasospasm[37]

- Respiratory failure
- Anaphylactic reactions

These symptoms are not only because of the mechanical embolism of the pulmonary artery, but also immune-mediated due to several cytokines, bradykinin, and so forth, which is quite similar to anaphylaxis.[38]

The clinical signs start with hypotension and fetal distress with a rapid onset; furthermore, dyspnea, coagulopathy, and seizures can occur. There is no specific management for AFE, but the full ICU setting can be needed to treat the patient, because CPR, mechanical ventilation, right heart therapy with nitrous oxide, and extracorporeal membrane oxygenation (ECMO) might be required.

In most cases, neurologic damage after AFE is common.[38]

Acute Respiratory Distress Syndrome in Pregnancy

The causes of ARDS in pregnant patients are multiple and can have obstetric and nonobstetric reasons (**Table 1**).

The definition of ARDS was revisited in 2011, known as the "the Berlin definition"[39] (**Table 2**).

Pathophysiology of ARDS is characterized by a severe inflammation of the lung with a dysfunction of the alveoli-capillary unit. This leads to an activation of proinflammatory mediators, flooding of protein-rich edema into the alveolus, and surfactant dysfunction.

Atelectasis and increase of pulmonary shunt follows, simultaneously fibrotic alterations of lung tissue begin.[40,41]

Treatment of ARDS in pregnancy follows the same guidelines as in nonpregnant patients, although there is a lack of data. Principles are lung-protective ventilation, adequate anti-infectious medication, and supportive therapy of sepsis syndrome.[42]

In more severe cases, prone positioning, administration of nitrous oxide, high-frequency oscillation ventilation, and ECMO therapy may be necessary.

ECMO therapy is more in focus to treat severe respiratory failure with refractory hypoxemia since the 2009 H1N1 pandemic. In a case series from Australia and New Zealand, pregnant or postpartum patients on ECMO had a better than expected outcome: 14.1% (9 patients) received ECMO therapy, 6 of them survived. Overall, there was a mortality of 11% (7 patients of 64).[43]

OXYGENATION GOAL IN PREGNANCY

As explained previously, hypoxia and acidosis are poorly tolerated in the fetus. The oxygenation goal in all kinds of respiratory failure should be a maternal SpO2 of 95% or a Pa_{O_2} of 70 mm Hg or higher. If this is not achieved with insufflation of oxygen, invasive or noninvasive ventilation is necessary.

Table 1 Causes of acute respiratory distress syndrome in pregnancy	
Obstetric	**Nonobstetric**
Aspiration	Pneumonia
Amniotic fluid embolism	Transfusion
(Pre)Eclampsia	Trauma
Septic abortion	Fat embolism
Hemorrhage	Cardiac pulmonary edema
Tocolytic induced pulmonary edema	

Table 2	
Acute respiratory distress syndrome Berlin definition	
Timing	One week since insult or worsening
Chest imaging	Bilateral infiltrates (no effusions, collapse, nodules)
Origin of edema	No cardiac origin, no fluid overload, evaluation with echocardiography
Oxygenation	Mild: Pao_2/Fio_2 200–300 mm Hg with PEEP $\geq$5 cmH_2O
	Moderate: Pao_2/Fio_2 100–200 mm Hg with PEEP >5 cmH_2O
	Severe: Pao_2/Fio_2 $\leq$100 with PEEP >5 cmH_2O

Abbreviation: PEEP, positive end expiratory pressure.
Adapted from Ranieri VM, Rubenfeld GD, Thompson BT, et al. Acute respiratory distress syndrome: the Berlin Definition. JAMA 2012;307(23):2530.

MECHANICAL VENTILATION IN PREGNANCY

All previously described diseases can result in severe respiratory failure and the need for mechanical ventilation.

Endotracheal Intubation

Due to the anatomic and physiologic changes in pregnancy described previously, intubation failure is 8 times more common than in nonpregnant patients.[44] Additionally, an increased risk of aspiration makes the intubation more difficult. Due to decreased oxygen reserve induced by decreased FRC and increase of oxygen consumption, intubation should be performed quickly with cricoid pressure without ventilation with a face mask (rapid sequence induction). Preoxygenation with 100% O_2 is essential. Because of delayed gastric emptying and increased abdominal pressure, the pregnant patient should be regarded as not fasting.

Equipment for difficult airway management and suctioning devices should be available immediately.

Ventilator Settings

There is a lack of studies dealing with prolonged mechanical ventilation in pregnancy. As a basic principle, as in nonpregnant patients, barotrauma and volutrauma ("stress and strain") of the lung should be avoided.[45]

Ventilation should be set regarding the recommendations of the ARDS network. One basic principle is the low-tidal-volume ventilation (4–6 mL/kg predicted body weight).[46]

The usual pressure limits of the common recommendation may not be fully applicable in pregnant patients because of the increased chest wall compliance and the higher abdominal pressure of the uterus.

Therefore, a higher peak inspiratory pressure and positive end expiratory pressure (PEEP) should be set in pregnant patients. Measurement of transpulmonary pressure at bedside could be a helpful tool and a promising approach in these patients.

Because pregnant patients are adapted to a lower $Paco_2$ with consecutive metabolic compensation and lower bicarbonate, further hyperventilation should be avoided to prevent impairment of uterine blood flow. $Paco_2$ should not be lower than 30 mm Hg.

Permissive hypercapnia with $Paco_2$ of 60 mm Hg seems to have no adverse effect on the fetus, but higher levels of CO_2 should be avoided. In delivery, a higher $Paco_2$ in the mother is associated with a higher APGAR than a lower $Paco_2$,[11,47] but a control of maternal pH is essential (goal 7.25–7.35).

Oxygenation goal should be a Pao_2 higher than 70 mm Hg to guarantee sufficient fetal oxygenation.

A head-up position and daily awaking trials and spontaneous breathing trials complete the ventilation management of pregnant patients.

Noninvasive Ventilation

In recent years, full awake, not sedated patients become more and more important to improve outcome in the ICU. Hence, the use of noninvasive ventilation (NIV) has increased to avoid intubation, the use of sedation drugs, and to reduce the incidence of delirium.

In pregnancy, NIV is often avoided because of the increased risk of aspiration due to increased abdominal pressure and lower esophagus sphincter tone. There is also a lack of data on this issue, but some case studies report a successful application.[48]

Most investigators emphasize the necessary experience in NIV therapy if used in pregnant patients. Patients should be alert, in a head-up position, and cooperative.

Sedation for Mechanical Ventilation

Most drugs that are used for sedation in the ICU are not safe in pregnancy and should be avoided.

- *Propofol* has sedative effects on the fetus. Due to its lipophilic characteristics, it easily passes the placenta. Adverse effects on the fetus depend on dosage and duration of administration, so short-term use, for example, for induction of anesthesia, seems not to harm the fetus.
- *Benzodiazepines* cross the placenta and may accumulate in the fetus. Therefore, long-term acting benzodiazepines, such as diazepam, should be avoided. In lorazepam and midazolam, this effect is less and the clinical impact is not clear. There is no experience with lormetazepam in pregnancy. All benzodiazepines can cause congenital malformations.[49]
- Long-acting *opioids* like fentanyl should not be used in pregnant patients, because their use is associated with neonatal respiratory depression and neurologic disorders. Short-acting opioids, such as remifentanil, seem to be safe in pregnancy and can be used particularly for NIV.
- *Nondepolarizing blocking agents* pass the placenta and thus prolonged use leads to respiratory failure of the fetus, but short-term effects are unlikely. However, in delivery, assisted ventilation of the newborn should be anticipated.
- *Dexmedetomidine*, a selective alpha-2-receptor agonist, passes the placenta minimally in comparison with clonidine.[50] Due to its rapid clearance and its sedating and analgesic effects, it can be an alternative drug for treatment of pregnant patients. In animal experiments, no adverse effect on the fetus emerged.[51]

Does Delivery Improve Respiratory Failure?

Indication for delivery is given if the fetus shows signs of hypoxemia:

- Bradycardia
- Lack of heart rate variability
- Late decelerations with contractions

Delivery is also indicated in illnesses that are maintained by pregnancy, such as HELLP syndrome (hemolysis, elevated liver enzym levels, low platelet count) or amniotic fluid syndrome; however, delivery is not indicated in every case of respiratory failure, because there is only a little improvement of oxygenation and a small change in compliance or PEEP requirement.[52,53]

In other conditions, such as pneumonia or ARDS, it is not clear if delivery improves respiratory failure. Hence, the indication for delivery should be an interdisciplinary decision among intensivist, obstetrician, and neonatologist.

REFERENCES

1. Vasquez DN, Estenssoro E, Canales HS, et al. Clinical characteristics and outcomes of obstetric patients requiring ICU admission. Chest 2007;131(3): 718–24.
2. Pollock W, Rose L, Dennis CL. Pregnant and postpartum admissions to the intensive care unit: a systematic review. Intensive Care Med 2010;36(9):1465–74.
3. Weinberger SE, Weiss ST, Cohen WR, et al. Pregnancy and the lung. Am Rev Respir Dis 1980;121(3):559–81.
4. Lapinsky SE. Cardiopulmonary complications of pregnancy. Crit Care Med 2005; 33(7):1616–22.
5. Soothill PW, Nicolaides KH, Rodeck CH, et al. Blood gases and acid-base status of the human second-trimester fetus. Obstet Gynecol 1986;68(2):173–6.
6. Hampl V, Jakoubek V. Regulation of fetoplacental vascular bed by hypoxia. Physiol Res 2009;58(Suppl 2):S87–93.
7. Assali NS. Dynamics of the uteroplacental circulation in health and disease. Am J Perinatol 1989;6(2):105–9.
8. Meschia G. Fetal oxygenation and maternal ventilation. Clin Chest Med 2011; 32(1):15–9, vii.
9. Polvi HJ, Pirhonen JP, Erkkola RU. The hemodynamic effects of maternal hypo- and hyperoxygenation in healthy term pregnancies. Obstet Gynecol 1995; 86(5):795–9.
10. Levinson G, Shnider SM, DeLorimier AA, et al. Effects of maternal hyperventilation on uterine blood flow and fetal oxygenation and acid-base status. Anesthesiology 1974;40(4):340–7.
11. Peng AT, Blancato LS, Motoyama EK. Effect of maternal hypocapnia v. eucapnia on the foetus during Caesarean section. Br J Anaesth 1972;44(11):1173–8.
12. Rigby FB, Pastorek JG. Pneumonia during pregnancy. Clin Obstet Gynecol 1996; 39(1):107–19.
13. Goodnight WH, Soper DE. Pneumonia in pregnancy. Crit Care Med 2005;33(10 Suppl):S390–7.
14. Sheffield JS, Cunningham FG. Community-acquired pneumonia in pregnancy. Obstet Gynecol 2009;114(4):915–22.
15. Munn MB, Groome LJ, Atterbury JL, et al. Pneumonia as a complication of pregnancy. J Matern Fetal Med 1999;8(4):151–4.
16. Madinger NE, Greenspoon JS, Ellrodt AG. Pneumonia during pregnancy: has modern technology improved maternal and fetal outcome? Am J Obstet Gynecol 1989;161(3):657–62.
17. Centers for Disease Control and Prevention (CDC). Influenza vaccination coverage among pregnant women: 2011-12 influenza season, United States. MMWR Morb Mortal Wkly Rep 2012;61:758–63.
18. Louie JK, Salibay CJ, Kang M, et al. Pregnancy and severe influenza infection in the 2013-2014 influenza season. Obstet Gynecol 2015;125(1):184–92.
19. Harger JH, Ernest JM, Thurnau GR, et al, National Institute of Child Health and Human Development, Network of Maternal-Fetal Medicine Units. Risk factors

and outcome of varicella-zoster virus pneumonia in pregnant women. J Infect Dis 2002;185(4):422–7.

20. Kwon HL, Triche EW, Belanger K, et al. The epidemiology of asthma during pregnancy: prevalence, diagnosis, and symptoms. Immunol Allergy Clin North Am 2006;26(1):29–62.

21. Tamási L, Horváth I, Bohács A, et al. Asthma in pregnancy–immunological changes and clinical management. Respir Med 2011;105(2):159–64.

22. Samuelson WM, Kopita JM. Management of the difficult asthmatic. Gastroesophageal reflux, sinusitis, and pregnancy. Respir Care Clin N Am 1995;1(2):287–308.

23. Gandhi S, Sun D, Park AL, et al. The pulmonary edema preeclampsia evaluation (PEPE) study. J Obstet Gynaecol Can 2014;36(12):1065–70.

24. Lamont RF. The pathophysiology of pulmonary oedema with the use of beta-agonists. BJOG 2000;107(4):439–44.

25. Waybright RA, Coolidge W, Johnson TJ. Treatment of clinical aspiration: a reappraisal. Am J Health Syst Pharm 2013;70(15):1291–300.

26. Brown HL, Hiett AK. Deep vein thrombosis and pulmonary embolism in pregnancy: diagnosis, complications, and management. Clin Obstet Gynecol 2010; 53(2):345–59.

27. Heit JA, Kobbervig CE, James AH, et al. Trends in the incidence of venous thromboembolism during pregnancy or postpartum: a 30-year population-based study. Ann Intern Med 2005;143(10):697–706.

28. Bates SM, Greer IA, Middeldorp S, et al, American College of Chest Physicians. VTE, thrombophilia, antithrombotic therapy, and pregnancy: antithrombotic therapy and prevention of thrombosis, 9th ed: American College of Chest Physicians Evidence-Based Clinical Practice Guidelines. Chest 2012;141(2 Suppl): e691S–736S.

29. Chan WS, Chunilal S, Lee A, et al. A red blood cell agglutination D-dimer test to exclude deep venous thrombosis in pregnancy. Ann Intern Med 2007;147(3): 165–70.

30. Marshall AL. Diagnosis, treatment, and prevention of venous thromboembolism in pregnancy. Postgrad Med 2014;126(7):25–34.

31. Turrentine MA, Braems G, Ramirez MM. Use of thrombolytics for the treatment of thromboembolic disease during pregnancy. Obstet Gynecol Surv 1995;50(7): 534–41.

32. Brown HL. Air embolism during pregnancy. Obstet Gynecol 2008;111(2 Pt 2): 481–2.

33. Kim CS, Liu J, Kwon JY, et al. Venous air embolism during surgery, especially cesarean delivery. J Korean Med Sci 2008;23(5):753–61.

34. Fildes J, Reed L, Jones N, et al. Trauma: the leading cause of maternal death. J Trauma 1992;32(5):643–5.

35. Mendez-Figueroa H, Dahlke JD, Vrees RA, et al. Trauma in pregnancy: an updated systematic review. Am J Obstet Gynecol 2013;209(1):1–10.

36. McDonnell NJ, Percival V, Paech MJ. Amniotic fluid embolism: a leading cause of maternal death yet still a medical conundrum. Int J Obstet Anesth 2013;22(4): 329–36.

37. Clark SL, Cotton DB, Gonik B, et al. Central hemodynamic alterations in amniotic fluid embolism. Am J Obstet Gynecol 1988;158(5):1124–6.

38. Clark SL, Hankins GD, Dudley DA, et al. Amniotic fluid embolism: analysis of the national registry. Am J Obstet Gynecol 1995;172(4 Pt 1):1158–67 [discussion: 1167–9].

39. Ranieri VM, Rubenfeld GD, Thompson BT, et al. Acute respiratory distress syndrome: the Berlin definition. JAMA 2012;307(23):2526–33.

40. Matthay MA, Ware LB, Zimmerman GA. The acute respiratory distress syndrome. J Clin Invest 2012;122(8):2731–40.
41. Ware LB, Matthay MA. The acute respiratory distress syndrome. N Engl J Med 2000;342(18):1334–49.
42. Dellinger RP, Levy MM, Rhodes A, et al, Pediatric Subgroup. Surviving sepsis campaign: international guidelines for management of severe sepsis and septic shock: 2012. Crit Care Med 2013;41(2):580–637.
43. ANZIC Influenza Investigators and Australasian Maternity Outcomes Surveillance System. Critical illness due to 2009 A/H1N1 influenza in pregnant and postpartum women: population based cohort study. BMJ 2010;340:c1279.
44. Munnur U, de Boisblanc B, Suresh MS. Airway problems in pregnancy. Crit Care Med 2005;33(10 Suppl):S259–68.
45. Slutsky AS, Ranieri VM. Ventilator-induced lung injury. N Engl J Med 2014; 370(10):980.
46. Campbell LA, Klocke RA. Implications for the pregnant patient. Am J Respir Crit Care Med 2001;163(5):1051–4.
47. Ivankovic AD, Elam JO, Huffman J. Effect of maternal hypercarbia on the newborn infant. Am J Obstet Gynecol 1970;107(6):939–46.
48. Allred CC, Matías Esquinas A, Caronia J, et al. Successful use of noninvasive ventilation in pregnancy. Eur Respir Rev 2014;23(131):142–4.
49. McElhatton PR. The effects of benzodiazepine use during pregnancy and lactation. Reprod Toxicol 1994;8(6):461–75.
50. Ala-Kokko TI, Pienimäki P, Lampela E, et al. Transfer of clonidine and dexmedetomidine across the isolated perfused human placenta. Acta Anaesthesiol Scand 1997;41(2):313–9.
51. Tariq M, Cerny V, Elfaki I, et al. Effects of subchronic versus acute in utero exposure to dexmedetomidine on foetal developments in rats. Basic Clin Pharmacol Toxicol 2008;103(2):180–5.
52. Tomlinson MW, Caruthers TJ, Whitty JE, et al. Does delivery improve maternal condition in the respiratory-compromised gravida? Obstet Gynecol 1998;91(1): 108–11.
53. Mabie WC, Barton JR, Sibai BM. Adult respiratory distress syndrome in pregnancy. Am J Obstet Gynecol 1992;167(4 Pt 1):950–7.

Management of Complex Cardiac Issues in the Pregnant Patient

Huayong Hu, MD[a],*, Ioana Pasca, MD[b]

KEYWORDS

- ICU management of cardiac disease during pregnancy • Fetal oxygenation
- Vasopressor effects on fetal oxygenation • Valvular heart disease during pregnancy
- Fetal monitoring

KEY POINTS

- Maternal hemodynamic optimization requires understanding of physiologic changes during pregnancy and fetal oxygenation in order to protect the wellbeing of the mother and her fetus.
- Most physiology research regarding the maternal and fetal impact of pharmacologic agents come from otherwise healthy animal studies. A few randomized trials involving healthy patients on treating maternal hypotension from neuraxial anesthesia exist. However, fetal outcome data from treating pregnant patients with severe reduction of cardiopulmonary reserve is lacking.
- Multiple fetal monitoring techniques can sample fetal peripheral oxygenation and pH but have poor correlation with cord blood gas measurements. This is due to complex fetal compensatory mechanisms that maintain central perfusion and oxygenation in the setting of decreased global fetal oxygen delivery.

INTRODUCTION

Peripartum heart disease ranges from gravid patients with congenital anomalies to pregnant women with myocardial infarction, dilated cardiomyopathy, and valvular disorders made worse by high-output physiology. The critical care management of these patients has limited evidence-based data, and even those conclusions are drawn from healthy animal models.

Cardiac disease in pregnancy accounts for 10% to 15% of maternal mortality, and 1% to 3% of pregnant women have heart disease.[1] Adverse cardiac outcomes have been reported in 11% of completed pregnancies in women with congenital heart

Disclosure: Authors have nothing to disclose.
[a] Department of Anesthesiology, Yale New Haven Hospital, New Haven, CT, USA; [b] Department of Anesthesiology, Loma Linda University Medical Center, Loma Linda, CA, USA
* Corresponding author.
E-mail addresses: Huayong.hu@gmail.com; huayong.hu@yale.edu

Crit Care Clin 32 (2016) 97–107
http://dx.doi.org/10.1016/j.ccc.2015.08.004
0749-0704/16/$ – see front matter © 2016 Elsevier Inc. All rights reserved.

criticalcare.theclinics.com

disease: the most common being congestive heart failure and arrhythmias.[2] Furthermore, premature delivery rates were high (16%), children were more frequently small for gestational age, fetal mortality was 4%, 15% had spontaneous miscarriages, and 5% had elective abortion.[2]

MANAGEMENT GOALS

There are 2 major goals in managing the critically ill pregnant patient: stabilization of maternal condition and maintaining fetal well-being. There is limited evidence through comparative studies for guidance in optimizing these 2 goals simultaneously. In order to better understand the fetal implications and to improve fetal conditions during maternal treatment, one must first understand the maternofetal physiology.

Maternal Physiology

Physiologic changes of pregnancy include increased uterine blood flow (UBF) from approximately 50 to 100 mL/min to 350 to 700 mL/min, requiring 12% of cardiac output in the third trimester.[3,4] Increased uterine perfusion is mediated by an increase in circulating blood volume: red blood cell mass increases by 20% to 30%, plasma volume increases by 45% to 55% with a relative anemia of pregnancy.[5] Furthermore, there is dilation of uterine vessels with an effective uterine arteriovenous shunt that helps decrease systemic vascular resistance (SVR). SVR decreases to 35% less than prepregnancy levels in the second trimester and to 20% less than baseline at term.[6] Cardiac output increases through the second trimester of pregnancy to 30% to 60% more than prepregnancy levels[7] and continues to increase during labor from sympathetic stimulation and autotransfusion from uterine contractions.

Pulmonary artery catheterization performed in healthy parturients 36 to 38 weeks pregnant and again at 11 to 13 weeks postpartum revealed a 43% increase in cardiac output during late pregnancy and a 17% increase in heart rate. Mean arterial pressure (MAP), central venous pressure, pulmonary capillary wedge pressure, and left ventricular stroke work index were not different antepartum compared with postpartum.[8] Immediately postpartum, circulating volume and cardiac output are further increased as vena caval compression is relieved, and UBF decreases. However, within 1 hour of delivery, heart rate and cardiac output returned to prelabor values, and by 24 hours, all hemodynamic variables had returned to prelabor baseline.[8]

Fetal Oxygenation

Disturbance in fetal oxygenation in the setting of maternal shock can quickly lead to fetal distress. It is critically important to understand the factors affecting fetal oxygenation and its interaction with the maternal shock state. Different causes of maternal shock require different interventions. For example, hypovolemic shock requires either fluid or blood replacement and correcting the underlying cause; septic shock requires early fluid and appropriate antibiotic administration, vasopressor support of vascular tone (norepinephrine, epinephrine, vasopressin, etc.), and source control of the infection; cardiogenic shock demands timely correction of the underlying cause of pump failure, including early revascularization, inotropic support to increase contractility, and even mechanical circulatory support to maintain cardiac output in severe refractory cases. A pregnant patient provides a unique challenge, which is the condition of the fetus during the course of treatment for the mother. Currently, there is no strong evidence with regard to how to optimize the condition of the fetus other than optimizing the condition of the mother. Extensive research effort has focused on the interaction between maternal UBF and fetal oxygenation, and vasopressor effects on UBF and fetal oxygenation. Because of the high-risk nature of this patient population and implications on fetal well-being, it is difficult, if not impossible, to conduct randomized controlled trials on these patients. Most research data have been gathered from animals (pregnant sheep), although some observational data from human patients exist.

The unique challenge in taking care of pregnant patients in shock centers on oxygenation of the fetus. The fetal heart provides circulation, but the function of the lungs is replaced by the placenta, where gas exchange occurs. Umbilical arteries carry the deoxygenated blood with high carbon dioxide content to the placenta, and the umbilical vein carries the oxygenated blood with lower CO_2 content back to the fetal heart. On the maternal side of the placenta, uterine arteries carry oxygenated maternal blood with low CO_2 content to the placenta, where maternal and fetal bloodstreams get into close proximity for gas exchange. Wilkening and Meschia[9] in their research on pregnant sheep demonstrated that a simple mathematical model could quantify the effect of uterine artery oxygen delivery (uterine artery blood flow × oxygen content) on fetal umbilical vein oxygen tension. This model was derived from the Fick principle, the oxyhemoglobin dissociation curve, and the relation between fetal oxygen consumption and uterine artery oxygen delivery. Their study provides several insights into fetal oxygenation: (1) Oxygenated maternal uterine artery blood provides the source of oxygen for her fetus. (2) There is a high level of baseline UBF/oxygen delivery compared with the threshold at which fetal metabolic acidemia begins to develop due to lack of oxygen supply. They reported the baseline uterine oxygen delivery to be 2 to 3 times of this threshold value. (3) Uterine artery oxygen delivery has 3 key components: blood flow, hemoglobin concentration, and oxygen saturation. A severe reduction in any of these 3 variables can compromise oxygen delivery to the fetus, and by inference, an increase in one variable could compensate for reduction in others. However, in their study, only uterine artery blood flow was varied experimentally.

PHARMACOLOGIC STRATEGIES
Vasopressor Effects on Uterine Artery Blood Flow and Fetal Oxygenation

Because vasopressor infusion is an important therapy to stabilize patients in the intensive care unit (ICU), much effort has been used in elucidating the effects of vasoactive drugs on UBF and fetal oxygenation. Not surprisingly, almost all experimental data are obtained from healthy animals. Dopamine and dobutamine are commonly used vasoactive agents with both vasoconstrictive and inotropic effects. Their effects on UBF and consequently on fetal oxygenation have been examined. One study demonstrated that both drugs decreased UBF in a linear dose-effect relationship in pregnant sheep.[10] A more recent study of sheep re-examined the issue of dobutamine's effect on fetal oxygenation with the hypothesis that it would decrease fetal oxygenation.[11] They found that with prolonged infusion (up to 60 minutes), maternal MAP decreased below baseline, thought to be due to the antagonistic effect of 3-O-methyldobutamine (a metabolite of dobutamine) at the αreceptors. Interestingly, they also found the maternal hemoglobin increased by about 50% during the infusion period. UBF showed an initial increase, but at the 60-minute time point, high-dose dobutamine at 10 µg/kg/min was associated with a slight reduction of UBF from baseline likely because of decreased MAP. Despite this slight decrease in UBF, fetal oxygenation was maintained above baseline value. The increase in maternal hemoglobin compensated for the slight decrease in UBF with an end result of increased oxygen delivery to the uterus. The increase in hemoglobin was most likely due to splenic contraction induced by dobutamine, leading to more circulating red blood cells. This study provides evidence that increasing hemoglobin can compensate for decreasing UBF in maintaining oxygen delivery to the fetus.

Another animal study compared the effects of bolus doses of epidural isoproterenol and epinephrine on UBF.[12] Low-dose epinephrine bolus via epidural catheter is commonly given to rule out intravenous placement of the catheter in labor epidurals. In the event of an inadvertent intravenous placement of the catheter, injection of epinephrine increases the maternal heart rate and blood pressure, which provides evidence for a misplaced catheter. This study showed that isoproterenol caused mild maternal hypotension with proportional decrease in UBF. On the other hand, epinephrine either maintained or increased maternal MAP but severely decreased UBF (down to 50% from baseline). This study provides evidence that increasing maternal blood pressure via a vasoactive agent could actually decrease UBF dramatically.

Norepinephrine is a commonly used vasoactive agent with strong vasoconstricting and mild inotropic effects. Laboring women have elevated epinephrine and norepinephrine levels, and the onset of labor analgesia is associated with a reduction in epinephrine but not norepinephrine levels. An in vitro study examining the effects of these 2 drugs on uterine arterioles showed that norepinephrine caused vasoconstriction of the arteriole. This vasoconstricting effect of norepinephrine was blunted by prazosin (an α blocker) as well as low-dose epinephrine (at physiologic concentrations found in laboring women). Epinephrine at the low physiologic concentrations caused mild vasodilation, but this vasodilating effect was completely blocked by propranolol (a β blocker). As epinephrine concentration increases, the predominant effect on the arterioles is vasoconstriction via α receptor activation. This article provides evidence that α receptor activation causes uterine arteriole vasoconstriction and β receptor stimulation causes uterine arteriole vasodilation.[13]

In a study by McGrath and colleagues,[14] the authors induced hypotension in gravid ewes by administering local anesthesia via epidural catheters causing vasodilation. They compared the effects of ephedrine (indirect activity at α and β receptor sites), phenylephrine (a pure α-receptor agonist), and saline placebo on maternal MAP, UBF, SVR, and uterine vascular resistance (UVR). In this study, epidurally administered local anesthesia decreased SVR, MAP, and UBF, while exerting no significant effect on UVR. In this setting of hypotension secondary to vasodilation, both ephedrine and phenylephrine were able to restore the maternal MAP, but only ephedrine returned UBF close to baseline. When compared with the saline placebo group, phenylephrine caused further reduction of UBF despite that hypotension and low UBF persisted in the saline placebo group. Ephedrine therefore has been the drug of choice to treat maternal hypotension caused by neuraxial anesthesia for laboring women, until recently other studies have shown more fetal acidosis is associated with ephedrine than phenylephrine in healthy laboring women.

In the studies on healthy women undergoing elective cesarean section with spinal anesthesia, ephedrine use was associated with higher fetal oxygen delivery as well as increased fetal production of CO_2, increased fetal consumption of O_2, lower fetal pH, and increased fetal lactate concentration. These potentially deleterious effects are not seen with phenylephrine use, even though it reduces uterine oxygen delivery.[15] Given the high safety margin of uterine oxygen delivery, fetal oxygenation does not appear to be endangered by treating hypotension secondary to neuraxial anesthesia with phenylephrine in healthy laboring women. It is unclear how this result translates to patients with severe cardiopulmonary disease, wherein decreased reserve exists in terms of uterine oxygen delivery and fetal oxygenation. In those patients, phenylephrine might worsen fetal hypoxemia and acidosis, but ephedrine's effect of increasing fetal metabolism and oxygen consumption due to adrenergic stimulation is likely undesirable in the setting of low fetal oxygen supply. On the other hand, adrenergic stimulation plays a vital compensatory role during acute fetal hypoxemia. A surge of catecholamine release redistributes fetal cardiac output and available oxygen to vital organs such as the brain, heart, and adrenal glands at the expense of fetal skin, lungs, kidneys, and gastrointestinal tract.[16] More data on the effects of these vasoactive drugs are needed in patients with limited reserve of uterine oxygen delivery (**Box 1**).

Pharmacologic Agents in Valvular Heart Disease

Atrial fibrillation in pregnant women with valvular disease is associated with thrombo-embolic disease, and besides rate control, these women must be anticoagulated. Per American Heart Association (AHA) guidelines, atrial fibrillation during pregnancy can be treated with β-blockers, digoxin, or a nondihydropyridine calcium channel blocker.[17] β-Blockers range from pregnancy risk class C to class D and continue to be a source of debate in obstetrics literature. A 2013 meta-analysis on first-trimester β-blocker use showed a possible trend toward cleft lip/palate, fetal cardio-vascular disease, and neural tube defects.[18] Atenolol, which was previously recommended in pregnancy, is now scheduled pregnancy class D. One study on

---

Box 1
Lessons learned from animal studies of vasopressors on uterine blood flow and fetal oxygenation

1. Maternal hypotension decreases UBF and therefore fetal oxygenation.

2. Restoring maternal MAP with vasoactive agents might be necessary to stabilize the mother, but it does not necessarily restore UBF or fetal oxygenation. In fact, they commonly cause reduction of UBF. Using a vasoconstrictor to restore MAP even in distributive shock has been shown to further decrease UBF compared with placebo.

3. As demonstrated by Wilkening and Meschia, the uterine oxygen delivery determines fetal oxygenation, and the 3 components of uterine oxygen delivery (uterine blood flow, hemoglobin, and oxygen saturation) are all important factors in the overall oxygen delivery. Therefore, increasing maternal hemoglobin should improve fetal oxygenation. The minimum hemoglobin at which to transfuse in the ICU has been steadily decreasing after studies have shown either no difference or improved outcome for the patients at lower hemoglobin. However, for pregnant ICU patients, the importance of maintaining fetal oxygenation in the setting of decreased UBF or oxygen saturation requires a unique consideration of their transfusion trigger.

4. Most studies of effects of vasopressors on UBF and fetal oxygenation are done in healthy animals and humans. As we have learned, normal uterine oxygen delivery has a large safety margin that ensures adequate fetal oxygen supply during periods of maternal distress. The study results have to be cautiously applied to patients with severe cardiopulmonary diseases, because these patients have reduced reserve in terms of uterine oxygen delivery.

5. It is a difficult balance to achieve between maintaining maternal stability while not compromising fetal oxygenation, and between maintaining fetal oxygen delivery while not stimulating fetal oxygen consumption.

6. There is a strong need for better fetal monitoring of oxygenation status. Extending from the research by Wilkening and Meschia, a simple bedside noninvasive monitor of uterine oxygen delivery could help assess the status of fetal oxygenation during the course of treatment for the mother. A new technology named photoacoustic imaging, which applies laser pulse to tissue and then detects the generated ultrasound signals, has the potential to measure blood flow and oxygen saturation in a blood vessel. It is however still in the research phase of development.

223 women with 312 pregnancies treated for hypertension comparing atenolol mono-therapy with other drug therapies found atenolol use to be associated with lower birth weight and a trend toward preterm delivery, with closer correlations if used earlier in pregnancy and continued for a longer duration.[19] Metoprolol, like atenolol, crosses the placenta and can be found in cord blood. A prospective controlled trial of metoprolol-hydralazine-treated hypertensive pregnant women versus no pharmaco-logic treatment found similar fetal outcomes for birth weight, fetal bradycardia, and hy-poglycemia.[20] Amiodarone is also pregnancy class D and has been associated with fetal hypothyroidism and neurodevelopmental delay.[21] Few studies are available for digitalis use during pregnancy.

NONPHARMACOLOGIC MANAGEMENT STRATEGIES
Valvular Heart Disease of Pregnancy

Pregnant women with valvular heart disease who require care by an intensivist will likely be women with severe refractory heart failure with multi-organ system involve-ment. Further complicating management, the complex maternal and fetal physiology will depend on adequate uterine perfusion and unknown baseline placental angiogen-esis. The treatment of decompensated heart failure in pregnancy continues to priori-tize maternal stabilization, which may optimize fetal oxygenation. Few studies are available to guide medication selection in terms of maternal and fetal outcomes.

One of the largest prospective outcomes study looked at 546 women with congen-ital (74% of patients) or acquired cardiac lesions (22% of patients).[22] About 13% of women in the study had adverse cardiac events, including pulmonary edema, sus-tained arrhythmias requiring therapy, stroke, cardiac arrest, or death. Symptoms were significantly more likely to occur if they had left ventricular ejection fraction less than 40%, left heart obstruction due to either an aortic valve area less than 1.5 cm^2 or a mitral stenosis with a valve area less than 2.0 cm^2, New York Heart As-sociation (NYHA) class II or higher, or if they had a history of heart failure, transient ischemic attack, or stroke. Women in the study with no additional risk factors had a 4% occurrence of adverse cardiac events, with one risk factor 27%, and 2 or more risk factors 67% occurrence. This study also evaluated fetal outcomes including pre-mature birth, intrauterine growth retardation, respiratory distress syndrome, intraven-tricular hemorrhage, and death, which were related to NYHA class II or greater or left heart obstruction due to significant mitral or aortic stenosis. Adverse fetal outcomes were also affected by smoking during pregnancy, anticoagulant use during preg-nancy, and multiple gestations.

Women with obstructive valvular lesions (mitral and aortic stenosis) are at risk for worsened functional status due to pregnancy-related increases in cardiac output, ventricular volume, transvalvular pressures, and decreased diastolic time. Pulmonary hypertension due to valvular lesions in pregnancy further worsens hemodynamic sta-bility and mortality. Furthermore, high-end diastolic volumes in obstructive valvular disease predisposes to arrhythmias, especially atrial fibrillation, which is poorly toler-ated and often requires cardioversion.

The survival of cardiopulmonary bypass (CPB) in pregnant patients has reached the levels of nonpregnant patients; however, fetal mortality continues to be reported at 20% to 29%. CPB decreases maternal MAP and pulsatile flow, which raises uteropla-cental vascular resistance and worsens hypoxia. Further uteroplacental hypoperfu-sion occurs during the cooling and rewarming phases of CPB, which induces uterine contractions with irreversible uterine contractions considered one of the most important predictors of fetal death. In ewe lambs, very deep hypothermia was associated with a reduction of fetal heart rate of 7 beats per minute for each degree of fetal cooling. During cooling, there was maintenance of a fetomaternal temperature gradient likely due to the high fetal cardiac output,[23] with some centers advocating the use of normothermic CPB.[24] Additional strategies used to minimize fetal risks include minimizing intraoperative blood loss, maintaining uterine displacement, minimizing CPB times, maintaining a high flow rate (>2.4 L/min/m^2), and MAP 70 to 75 mm Hg.[24]

Mitral stenosis in pregnant women is most commonly due to rheumatic heart disease, endocarditis, or a congenital abnormality.[25] Women presenting with severe heart failure due to mitral stenosis may have failed medical management with furosemide, digoxin, or β-blockers. For patients refractory to medical therapy, percutaneous balloon mitral valvuloplasty may temporarily enlarge the mitral valve to allow continuation of pregnancy. A retrospective study comparing mitral valve commissurotomy and percutaneous balloon mitral valvuloplasty for women with severe mitral stenosis and heart failure showed similar maternal status postoperatively with significantly better fetal outcomes in the percutaneous group. Percutaneous repair was associated with a 4.8% fetal mortality compared with a 37.9% fetal mortality in the open repair group.[26] Therefore, American College of Cardiology (ACC)/AHA guidelines suggest pregnant patients with mitral stenosis and severe symptomatic heart failure could reasonably have percutaneous repair, and if percutaneous mitral valve repair cannot be done in pregnant patients with severe refractory heart failure, open commisurotomy might also be reasonable.[25]

Mitral regurgitation in pregnant women is most commonly due to mitral valve prolapse and is generally tolerated because of the low SVR state of pregnancy, which decreases regurgitant volume. Other common causes of mitral regurgitation include rheumatic heart disease (less likely in developed countries) and myxomatous degeneration due to connective tissue disorders. Hypertrophic cardiomyopathy and dilated cardiomyopathy can also enlarge the mitral annulus leading to functional mitral regurgitation. There have also been reports of acute mitral regurgitation due to torn chordae tendineae from myocardial infarction and perforated valve leaflets from endocarditis.

Associated with angina, syncope, and dyspnea, aortic stenosis in pregnant women is most commonly caused by congenital anomalies.[27] For aortic stenosis, there are no studies comparing percutaneous versus open aortic valve repair in pregnant patients with severe heart failure, but a case report showed good outcomes in 2 women with successful balloon dilatation of the aortic valve in the second trimester of pregnancy with good fetal outcomes.[28] Open repair of aortic valvulopathies continues to be associated with poor fetal outcomes. A study published in 2015 presenting 11 women in their second trimester of pregnancy with severe aortic stenosis and aortic regurgitation that underwent aortic surgery and CPB between 2004 and 2013 had a 27% rate of fetal mortality within 1 week of surgery. The surgery was performed using normothermia at 36°C with pulsatile perfusion to maintain MAPs of 70 mm Hg, avoidance of vasoconstrictors to avoid decreases in uterine perfusion, avoidance of circulatory arrest, maintenance of hemoglobin greater than 9 g/dL, and serial Doppler fetal ultrasonography of the umbilical and middle cerebral arterial resistance to monitor and improve fetal oxygenation.[29] However, even with these treatment strategies, fetal mortality after CPB remained similar to historical figures for fetal death related to CPB of 15% to 30%.[30] The remaining fetuses were delivered at term and were doing well at a mean follow-up of 4.2 years.

Decreased SVR of pregnancy will likely reduce regurgitant flow and left ventricular end diastolic volume in aortic regurgitation. Of patients who present with acute severe aortic regurgitation, it may be related to dilated aortic root due to connective tissue disease like Marfan or previous endocarditis. Symptomatic aortic regurgitation in pregnancy presenting to the intensivist is most likely due to acute regurgitation in which left ventricular enlargement and accommodation of volume has not occurred. Patients with Marfan syndrome are specifically at increased risk for acute aortic regurgitation due to arterial wall distension, aortic dissection, and aortic root dilation. For type A ascending aortic dissections during the first or second trimester, urgent surgical repair is recommended by the 2010 ACC/AHA/American Thoracic Society guidelines, and during the third trimester, type A dissections should be treated with urgent cesarean section followed by aortic repair.[31]

For patients with severe cardiogenic shock unresponsive to medical management and who are not candidates for valvular repair, there are not sufficient data to comment on the use of intra-aortic balloon pump (IABP), extracorporeal membrane oxygenation (ECMO), or continuous-flow left ventricular assist devices (LVAD). These devices have been attempted in critically ill women with peripartum cardiomyopathy, and one case series presented 2 women who had an IABP inserted before cesarean delivery. One of the women was weaned off IABP after 4 days and the other required LVAD to transplant with good long-term outcome.[32] One obstacle of ECMO in pregnancy is decreased venous drainage due to uterocaval compression by the gravid uterus with the need for uterine displacement, emergent delivery, or placement of additional venous cannulas.[33] The use of mechanical circulatory support in pregnant women with cardiogenic shock remains to be determined on a case-by-case basis guided by physiology.

FETAL EVALUATION

The pregnant patient in cardiogenic shock may present with peripartum cardiomyopathy, acute myocardial infarction, worsening chronic heart failure, or worsening chronic congenital anomalies. The framework of the pregnant ewe fetal physiology studies is encouraging for future studies of human fetal oxygenation, but currently there are only indirect conclusions that can be used in pregnant women with cardiogenic shock. Regardless of the cause, the balance between improving cardiac output with vasopressor agents and worsening UBF is difficult and further complicated by limited ability to monitor oxygenation of vital fetal organs.

Ideally, fetal monitors would allow quantification of fetal perfusion and oxygenation, but changes in fetal heart rate, fetal pulse oximetry, and measurement of fetal scalp pH have correlated poorly with umbilical cord blood acid-base status because complex fetal compensatory mechanisms can compensate until late in hypoxemia by preferentially shunting blood to the heart and brain. A 2008 multicenter prospective randomized controlled study including more than 3000 patients showed no difference in fetal metabolic acidosis when fetal scalp pH was compared with fetal scalp lactate, although smaller samples were required for lactate.[34] In 2014, Chandraharan[35] further explained that fetal scalp acidosis does not characterize central hypoperfusion, but instead, it is a marker of peripheral hypoperfusion due to regulatory mechanisms that shunt blood from peripheral organs like skin to central organs. In a Cochrane meta-analysis, fetal pulse oximetry was not shown to decrease the rate of cesarean section, and one study in the meta-analysis showed a higher rate of cesarean section when fetal pulse oximetry was used.[36] Similar to fetal scalp pH, fetal pulse oximetry measures peripheral oxygenation. There have been new hopes that fetal electrocardiogram monitoring with ST-waveform analysis may evaluate central fetal hypoxia. The rationale is that in compensated fetal hypoxia, the fetal heart can remain adequately oxygenated. When fetal myocardium is deprived of oxygen, there can be ST segment changes, which indicate failure of compensatory centralization of perfusion/oxygenation and impending fetal demise.[37] Although it is a step in the right direction toward monitoring central fetal oxygenation, clinical trials so far have shown mixed results.

The timing of fetal delivery should not delay maternal stabilization; however, fetal delivery may improve maternal hemodynamics and may allow for more invasive procedures like LVAD, IABP, and possibly ECMO if indicated.

DISCUSSION

The pregnant patient with severe cardiac issues may present with peripartum cardiomyopathy, acute myocardial infarction, worsening chronic heart failure, or worsening chronic congenital anomalies. The framework of the pregnant ewe fetal physiology studies is encouraging for future studies of human fetal oxygenation, but currently there are only indirect conclusions that can be used in pregnant women with cardiogenic shock. Maternal hemoglobin, oxygen saturation, and cardiac output impact fetal perfusion, although complex fetal compensation mechanisms, limit the specificity fetal monitoring.

REFERENCES

1. Huisman CM, Zwart JJ, Roos-Hesselink JW, et al. Incidence and predictors of maternal cardiovascular mortality and severe morbidity in the Netherlands: a prospective cohort study. PLoS One 2013;8(2):e56494.
2. Drenthen W, Pieper PG, Roos-Hesselink JW, et al, ZAHARA Investigators. Outcome of pregnancy in women with congenital heart disease: a literature review. J Am Coll Cardiol 2007;49:2303–11.
3. Edman CD, Toofanian A, MacDonald PC, et al. Placental clearance rate of maternal plasma androstenedione through placental estradiol formation: an indirect method of assessing uteroplacental blood flow. Am J Obstet Gynecol 1981; 141(8):1029–37.
4. Thaler I, Manor D, Itskovitz J, et al. Changes in uterine blood flow during human pregnancy. Am J Obstet Gynecol 1990;162:121–5.
5. Longo LD. Maternal blood volume and cardiac output during pregnancy: a hypothesis of endocrinologic control. Am J Phys 1983;245(5 Pt 1):R720–9.
6. Stoelting RK, Hines RL, Marschall KE, editors. Chapter 26 pregnancy-associated diseases. Stoelting's anesthesia and co-existing disease. 6th edition. Philadelphia: Saunders; 2012. p. 559.
7. Robson SC, Dunlop W, Boys RJ. Serial study of factors influencing changes in cardiac output during human pregnancy. Am J Phys 1989;256(4 pt 2):H1060–5.
8. Clark SL, Cotton DB, Lee W, et al. Central hemodynamic assessment of normal term pregnancy. Am J Obstet Gynecol 1989;161(6 pt 1):1439–42.
9. Wilkening R, Meschia G. Fetal oxygen uptake, oxygenation, and acid-base balance as a function of uterine blood flow. Am J Phys 1983;244(6):H749–55.
10. Fishburne J, Meis J, Urban B, et al. Vascular and uterine responses to dobutamine and dopamine in the gravid ewe. Am J Obstet Gynecol 1980;137:944.
11. Butler E, Moon P, Gleed R, et al. The effects of maternal plasma dobutamine levels on fetal oxygenation in anaesthetized sheep. Vet Anaesth Analg 2001; 28:34–41.
12. Marcus M, Vertommen J, Aken H, et al. Hemodynamic effects of intravenous isoproterenol versus epinephrine in the chronic maternal-fetal sheep preparation. Anesth Analg 1996;82:1023–6.

13. Segal S, Wang S. The effect of maternal catecholamines on the caliber of gravid uterine microvessels. Anesth Analg 2008;106:888–92.
14. McGrath J, Chestnut D, Vincent R, et al. Ephedrine remains the vasopressor of choice for treatment of hypotension during ritodrine infusion and epidural anesthesia. Anesthesiology 1994;80:1073–81.
15. Kee N, Lee A, Khaw K, et al. A randomized double-blinded comparison of phenylephrine and ephedrine infusion combinations to maintain blood pressure during spinal anesthesia for cesarean delivery: the effects on fetal acid-base status and hemodynamic control. Anesth Analg 2008;107:1295–302.
16. Jensen A, Garnier Y, Berger R. Dynamics of fetal circulatory responses to hypoxia and asphyxia. Eur J Obstet Gynecol Reprod Biol 1999;84:155–72.
17. Fuster V, Ryden L, Cannom D, et al. 2006 ACC/AHA/ESC guidelines for the management of patients with atrial fibrillation—executive summary a report of the American College of Cardiology/American Heart Association task force on practice guidelines and the European Society of Cardiology Committee for practice guidelines (writing committee to revise the 2001 guidelines for the management of patients with atrial fibrillation): developed in collaboration with the European Heart Rhythm Association and the Heart Rhythm Society. Circulation 2006;114: 700–52.
18. Yakoob MY, Bateman BT, Ho E, et al. The risk of congenital malformations associated with exposure to β-blockers early in pregnancy. Hypertension 2013;62: 375–81.
19. Lydakis C, Lip GY, Beevers M, et al. Atenolol and fetal growth in pregnancies complicated by hypertension. Am J Hypertens 1999;12:541.
20. Hogstedt S, Lindeberg S, Axelsson O, et al. A prospective controlled trial of metoprolol-hydralazine treatment in hypertension during pregnancy. Acta Obstet Gynecol Scand 1985;64(6):505–10.
21. Bartalena L, Bogazzi F, Braverman LE, et al. Effects of amiodarone administration during pregnancy on neonatal thyroid function and subsequent neurodevelopment. J Endocrinol Invest 2001;24:116–30.
22. Siu SC, Sermer M, Colman JM, et al. Prospective multicenter study of pregnancy outcomes in women with heart disease. Circulation 2001;104:515–21.
23. Pardi G, Ferrari M, Iorio F, et al. The effect of maternal hypothermic cardiopulmonary bypass on fetal lamb temperature, hemodynamics, oxygenation, and acid-base balance. J Thorac Cardiovasc Surg 2004;127:1728–34.
24. John A, Gurley F, Schaff H, et al. Cardiopulmonary bypass during pregnancy. Ann Thorac Surg 2011;91:1191–6.
25. Nishimura RA, Otto CM, Bonow RO, et al. 2014 AHA/ACC guideline for the management of patients with valvular heart disease: executive summary. J Am Coll Cardiol 2014;63(22):2438–88.
26. De Souza JA, Martinez EE, Ambrose JA, et al. Percutaneous balloon mitral valvuloplasty in comparison with open mitral valve commissurotomy for mitral stenosis during pregnancy. J Am Coll Cardiol 2001;37:900–3.
27. Reimold SC, Rutherford JD. Valvular heart disease in pregnancy. N Engl J Med 2003;349:52–9.
28. Banning AP, Person JF, Hall RJ. Role of balloon dilatation of the aortic valve in pregnant patients with severe aortic stenosis. Br Heart J 1993;70:544–5.
29. Yates MT, Soppa G, Smelt J, et al. Perioperative management and outcomes of aortic surgery during pregnancy. J Thorac Cardiovasc Surg 2015;149(2):607–10.
30. Lao T, Sermer M, MaGee L, et al. Congenital aortic stenosis and pregnancy – a reappraisal. Am J Obstet Gynecol 1993;169:540–5.

31. Hiratzka LF, Bakris GL, Beckman JA, et al. 2010 ACCF/AHA/AATS/ACR/ASA/ SCA/SCAI/SIR/STS/SVM guidelines for the diagnosis and management of patients with thoracic aortic disease: a report of the American College of Cardiology Foundation/American Heart Association Task Force on practice guidelines, American Association for Thoracic Surgery, American College of Radiology, American Stroke Association, Society of Cardiovascular Anesthesiologists, Society for Cardiovascular Angiography and Interventions, Society of Interventional Radiology, Society of Thoracic Surgeons, and Society for Vascular Medicine. Circulation 2010;121(13):e266.

32. Gavaert S, Belleghem YV, Bouchez S, et al. Acute and critically ill peripartum cardiomyopathy and 'bridge to' therapeutic options: a single center experience with intra-aortic balloon pump, extra corporeal membrane oxygenation and continuous-flow left ventricular assist devices. Crit Care 2011;15:R93.

33. Grasselli G, Bombino M, Patroniti N, et al. Use of extracorporeal respiratory support during pregnancy: a case report and literature review. ASAIO J 2012;58: 281–4.

34. Wiberg-Itzel E, Lipponer C, Norman M, et al. Determination of pH or lactate in fetal scalp blood in management of intrapartum fetal distress: randomized controlled multicentre trial. BMJ 2008;336:1284.

35. Chandraharan E. Fetal scalp blood sampling during labour: is it a useful diagnostic test or a historical test that no longer has a place in modern clinical obstetrics? BJOG 2014;121:1056–62.

36. East CE, Begg L, Colditz PB, et al. Fetal pulse oximetry for fetal assessment in labour. Cochrane Database Syst Rev 2014;(10):CD004075.

37. Chandraharan E, Sabaratnam A. Electronic fetal heart rate monitoring in current and future practice. J Obstet Gynecol India 2008;58(2):121–30.

Trauma Management of the Pregnant Patient

Amie Lucia, DO[a], Susan E. Dantoni, MD[b,c],*

KEYWORDS

- Trauma • Pregnant patient • Management • Fetus

KEY POINTS

- Trauma is a leading cause of nonobstetric maternal and fetal mortality.
- Pregnant patients should be treated systematically like all other trauma patients, but often standard trauma principles are deviated from when caring for a pregnant trauma patient.
- Education of at-risk pregnant patients can make a large impact on decreasing traumatic morbidity and mortality in this population and even preventing injuries.

INTRODUCTION

In 1 way or another pregnancy affects us all, whether that the development and birth of your own child, a close friend's, or a family member's. It would be wonderful if all of these experiences were guaranteed to be uncomplicated, but the pregnant woman is not exempt from anything in life, including trauma. Trauma continues to be a leading cause of maternal and fetal mortality worldwide.

When entering the trauma bay with a pregnant patient, it is fair to say that the stakes are immediately raised. Identifying the pregnant trauma patient will not always be easy, so it is imperative to test for pregnancy in all women of childbearing age. Pregnancy is not always detectable by physical examination, for example, in the early trimesters or in the setting of morbid obesity.

Once the pregnant patient is identified, not only does the provider have to consider 2 patients, but also understand the multiple anatomic and physiologic changes that occur during pregnancy and how to appropriately treat this subgroup of the population. The early establishment of a multidisciplinary team of individuals is imperative. These teams may often include an emergency medicine physician, trauma surgeon, obstetrician, critical care intensivist, and neonatologist. Although the treatment of

Nothing to disclose.
[a] SUNY Upstate Medical University, 750 E Adams street, Syracuse, NY 13210, USA; [b] Bellevue Women's Center/Ellis Hospital, Schenectady, New York, USA; [c] Department OB/GYN, Albany Medical College, 47 New Scotland Ave, Albany, NY 12208, USA
* Corresponding author.
E-mail address: obdocsue@aol.com

the mother precedes that of the fetus, a rule to keep in mind in these difficult situations is that what is good for the mother is almost always good for the fetus.

EPIDEMIOLOGY

Approximately 7% of pregnancies in the United States are affected by trauma and this is reported to be the leading cause of nonobstetric maternal and fetal mortality.[1,2] Falls, domestic violence, and motor vehicle crashes (MVCs) are the most common mechanisms of injury encountered in pregnant patients, whereas the most common causes of maternal mortality are penetrating trauma and MVCs.[3]

In a retrospective analysis of 321 pregnant trauma patients, blunt trauma was noted to be 10 times more common than penetrating trauma. However, maternal mortality was noted to be higher in the penetrating trauma group (7%) than the blunt trauma group (2%). The fetal mortality difference in penetrating and blunt trauma was even more pronounced at 73% and 10%, respectively.[4] Penetrating trauma should immediately raise concern for impending fetal demise.

According to US Centers for Disease Control and Prevention there are just over 4 million births reported yearly in the United States[5]; if 7% of them are affected by trauma, this totals just about 300,000 pregnant individuals affected by trauma in the United States alone per year. This is a significant number and being knowledgeable on the appropriate care for these patients is essential.

ANATOMY AND PHYSIOLOGY OF PREGNANCY
Anatomic Considerations

Throughout the pregnancy, as the fetus grows the uterus gradually ascends through the abdominal cavity, being limited to the pelvis for only the first 12 weeks. It reaches the umbilicus around week 20 and peaks at the costal margin between weeks 34 and 38. This leads to the gradual displacement of intraabdominal organs from their usual landmarks. During the first trimester, the fetus remains protected by the bony pelvis and a thick-walled uterus; however, this changes in the second and third trimester. As the fetus grows, it becomes the most anterior structure in the abdomen and is only protected by the soft tissue of the abdominal wall and the thinning uterine wall, leaving it as well as the uterus and placenta more vulnerable to injury. The enlarging uterus bestows protection to the maternal organs by pushing the bowel cephalad and encasing it by the lower rib cage and lying anterior to the retroperitoneal organs.

The uterus and placenta provide a new threat similar to solid organ injury in that they can lead to a significant amount of rapid blood loss causing hemorrhagic shock from a source that is difficult to identify visually. Other anatomic changes to consider include the slight widening of the pubic symphysis and an altered center of balance, leading to an increased predisposition to falls. Women in their third trimester have been shown to have a decrease in postural stability.[6] This may be one of the reasons women are more susceptible to trauma in the later stages of pregnancy.

Cardiovascular Physiology

In the pregnant patient, there is a greater circulating blood volume for 2 major reasons. First, there is systemic vasodilation and decreased peripheral vascular resistance, which can be seen as early as 5 weeks into pregnancy and is likely augmented by increases in progesterone and estrogen. This is accompanied by the growth and maturation of the placenta, a large vascular organ, which leads to a larger overall volume of distribution for circulating blood.[7] The vasodilation and increased volume of distribution results in an increased cardiac output, which can be up to 45% greater than normal. In multiple gestation pregnancies, this number can be even greater and can lead left atrial dilation representative of volume overload.[8]

The changes in vital signs during pregnancy are similar to those seen in the early stages of shock and should be evaluated cautiously. Heart rate during pregnancy is often increased by 10 to 20 bpm, most significantly in the third trimester. It is also common for the blood pressure of pregnant patients to be lower than that of their prepregnancy values. However, do not be misled into attributing tachycardia or hypotension in the pregnant trauma patient to normal physiologic changes until a thorough workup for traumatic injury is complete.[7] One of the immediate interventions to perform on the pregnant trauma patient in the later stages of pregnancy presenting with hypotension is placing them in the left lateral decubitus position to relieve the pressure of the gravid uterus from compressing the vena cava and decreasing preload to the heart.

Hematology

As stated, the circulatory volume is increased in a pregnant patient, which is represented by an increase in both plasma volume as well as red cell mass. However, the plasma volume increase is proportionally greater than that of the red cell mass, leading to the physiologic anemia of pregnancy.[7] These changes are accompanied by an increase in white blood cells as well as a relative hypercoaguable state that is multifactorial and not understood fully. This state becomes of further importance in the setting of massive hemorrhage or infection secondary to trauma because pregnant patients are predisposed to consumptive coagulapathies such as disseminated intravascular coagulation (DIC).[9] DIC can be diagnosed by measuring elevated serum levels of fibrin degradation products and D-dimers in the setting of relatively low fibrinogen levels. However, it is important to remember that the D-dimer level is often increased in trauma and fibrinogen levels are often increased in pregnancy. These laboratory values should be accompanied by a clinical picture of bleeding and thrombosis to make the diagnosis of DIC.

Respiratory Physiology

As the fetus grows and takes over more real estate in the abdomen, the diaphragm is pushed cephalad and the thoracic volume would decrease if there were no compensatory mechanism. However, the thoracic cavity is able to compensate. The rib cage makes some temporary adjustments by increasing the anterior–posterior as well and lateral diameters to increase the intrathoracic volume. This increased thoracic volume along with an increased basal respiratory rate and decreased residual volume allows the mother to respond to increased metabolic demands of pregnancy by increasing her overall tidal volume and minute ventilation.[10]

Gastrointestinal Physiology

Gastric emptying is often delayed, especially in the later stages of pregnancy. This is owing to displacement of and compression on the stomach by the enlarging uterus. This, accompanied by decreased esophageal sphincter competency secondary to increased levels of progesterone, places the pregnant patient at high risk for an aspiration event. Rapid sequence intubation and nasogastric tube decompression should always be considered in pending respiratory failure. Pregnancy is also associated with a state of cholestasis, which leads to a higher risk of biliary colic and acute cholecystitis in these patients (**Table 1**).

Table 1	
Anatomic and physiologic changes during pregnancy	
Change	**Description**
Uterine growth	At 20 wk, the fundal height is at the level of the umbilicus.
Cardiovascular	Systemic vasodilation, decreased peripheral vascular resistance, greater volume of distribution owing to placenta, increased cardiac output, increased heart rate, decreased blood pressure.
Hematology	Increased plasma volume, increased red cell mass, anemia, elevated white blood cell count, hypercoaguable state, elevated fibrinogen.
Respiratory	Increased respiratory rate, decreased residual volume, increased tidal volume, increased minute ventilation.
Gastrointestinal	Delayed gastric emptying, decreased esophageal sphincter competency, cholestasis.

ASSESSMENT AND MANAGEMENT
Primary Survey

The provider should adhere to the normal algorithm of evaluating and treating a trauma patient with a few adjuncts. It is essential to begin with the primary survey, ensuring that an airway is established and that there is sufficient ventilation and circulating blood volume for adequate oxygenation of the mother and fetus.[11] Volume and blood resuscitation should be anticipated and expeditious because signs of maternal and especially fetal distress may not be present until about one-third of the maternal blood volume is lost. Log rolling the patient to the left lateral decubitus position should be immediately considered in the hypotensive pregnant trauma patient to relieve pressure from the vena cava and increase central venous blood return.

Secondary Survey

A thorough obstetric history should be taken in addition to the routine history obtained from the trauma patient followed by a head to toe physical examination. A complete physical examination should include a pelvic examination to identify vaginal bleeding, ruptured membranes, or a bulging perineum. Adjunctive imaging including x-rays and the Focused Assessment with Sonography in Trauma examination should be performed as indicated in nonpregnant patients. As detailed in the section Radiology, obtaining imaging with ionizing radiation should not be delayed for potential concerns for the fetus.

Focused Assessment with Sonography in Trauma examinations are useful in pregnancy and most studies have been able to report a sensitivity of approximately 80% and a specificity of 100% for detecting major abdominal injury.[12] There is a small amount of physiologic free fluid in the pelvis during pregnancy; however, this is far too small to be detected by a conventional Focused Assessment with Sonography in Trauma examination and all fluid visualized should be considered pathologic.

In addition to standard blood work, a Kleihauer–Betke test should be obtained for patients in their second or third trimester to determine if there is any fetal blood in the maternal circulation. If positive, Rh-negative mothers should be treated with Rh-immune globulin to prevent sensitization to Rh antigens present in fetal blood.[11] This measure will decrease the chance of hemolytic disease of the newborn. However, using the Kleihauer–Betke test alone to detect significant maternal–fetal hemorrhage that would lead to fetal distress is controversial. Fetal heart rate monitoring remains the best way we have at this time to detect fetal distress. It is also helpful to monitor the hemodynamic and perfusion status of the mother, because maternal hypoperfusion or hypoxia is an indicator for fetal hypoperfusion and hypoxia, albeit a late sign. It may be more judicious to use fetal distress on a fetal heart rate monitor as an early marker of maternal hypovolemia.

PREGNANCY-ASSOCIATED PATHOLOGY

The pregnant trauma patient remains subject to the list of pathologic conditions that can affect all pregnant patients and it is important for providers to be familiar with these conditions. It is not unlikely that some of these disorders predispose these patients to a traumatic accident such as a fall or MVC by altering their sensorium.

Preeclampsia and Eclampsia

Preeclampsia is defined by new-onset hypertension in the setting of pregnancy, with a systolic pressure of greater than 140 mm Hg or a diastolic pressure of greater than 90 mm Hg. Patients often present with symptoms of headaches, peripheral edema, and abdominal pain. Laboratory values should be evaluated for proteinuria, elevated transaminases, and thrombocytopenia. Although patients with mild preeclampsia can be managed expectantly, severe preeclampsia is a state of poor placental perfusion, which should be optimized by resuscitation and definitive management, which is delivery of the fetus. Magnesium sulfate infusion should be initiated to prevent transition to eclampsia, which is hallmarked by development of seizures.[13] A high index of suspicion for this etiology of altered mental status in the trauma patient is essential, because this diagnosis could easily be overlooked as the precursor for the traumatic event.

Hemolysis, Elevated Liver Enzymes, and Low Platelets Syndrome

A life-threatening obstetric complication associated with preeclampsia and defined by Hemolysis, Elevated Liver enzymes and Low Platelets syndrome. Laboratory values are notable for elevated lactate dehydrogenase, elevated bilirubin levels, elevated transaminases, low platelets, and the presence of schistocytes. This condition, like preeclampsia, is ultimately treated by the delivery of the fetus and placenta.[13]

Amniotic Fluid Embolism

The incidence and mortality of amniotic fluid embolism varies widely throughout the literature and different populations. The most likely time of occurrence is intrapartum or immediately post partum and it is clinically characterized by the sudden onset of dyspnea, hypoxia and profound hypotension. Bedside echocardiogram can reveal right heart strain and or failure as well as increased pulmonary artery pressures. This is truly a clinical diagnosis of exclusion and treatment measures are limited to supportive care in an intensive care unit. Of patients with amniotic fluid embolisms, 50%will progress to develop DIC. A high index of suspicion to rapidly diagnose and initiate treatment of DIC could be lifesaving.[13]

INJURY PREVENTION

The main focus in the effort to decrease maternal and fetal morbidity and mortality with regard to trauma is injury prevention and maternal education, especially for pregnant patients with increased risk. A retrospective study in *The Journal of Women's Health* identified characteristics that were more common in mothers who reported injury. In this particular study, these characteristics included age less than 18 years, alcohol use, smoking, epilepsy, and employment.[14] Data from the American College of

Surgeon's National Trauma Data Bank identified young minority women at greater risk for traumatic injury during pregnancy.[15] Although these risk factors are not all modifiable, they help to characterize at risk populations that may benefit from more extensive education and counseling. As newer databases become more robust, including the National Violent Death Reporting System from the Centers for Disease Control and Prevention as well as the National Trauma Data Bank from the American College of Surgeons, we may be able to more accurately target women at risk for trauma during pregnancy.

Seatbelt Use

MVCs are among the leading causes of maternal and fetal injury and mortality in the United States. Seatbelt use in pregnant patients is among the most extensively studied modifiable risk factors. Lack of restraint use in pregnancy has been associated repeatedly with increased morbidity and mortality in both the mother and the fetus. However, women often report that they were not counseled on the benefits of seatbelt use during pregnancy.

The death of a fetus secondary to an MVC occur at a rate of 2.3 deaths per 100,000 live births, with a trend toward teenage pregnancies being at greater risk.[16] Adverse fetal outcomes in MVCs have been associated with higher crash severity, more severe maternal injury, and lack of proper seat belt use.[17] Wearing a seatbelt while pregnant has been demonstrated in simulations to reduce pressure exerted on the abdomen during impact in an MVC.[18] This is likely because the restraint prevents contact of the abdomen with the steering wheel. Wearing a seatbelt while pregnant can reduce the risk of fetal and maternal mortality in the setting of MVCs.[19,20]

Domestic Violence

Domestic violence or intimate partner violence is, unfortunately, among the most common causes of trauma in pregnancy. The incidence has been studied extensively and varies greatly among different populations ranging from 1% to 57%.[2] A study that reviewed the charts of 176,845 pregnant women in Massachusetts determined that women who presented with intentional injury, as well as substance abuse and mental illness, had a significantly higher rate of both low birth weight as well as preterm birth.[21]

Risk factors for intimate partner violence have been identified and include substance abuse, low socioeconomic status, limited education, unintended pregnancy, and a history of violence in previous close relationships.[2] Often, victims of domestic violence are unwilling to leave their current situation or report abuse because they depend on their partner both financially and emotionally. Health care providers should be proactive on identifying patients at risk and providing them with information on support groups and programs within the community.

RADIOLOGY

There is widespread concern with regard to the theoretic adverse outcomes of exposing a fetus to radiation that is routinely used in the workup of a trauma patient. This concern can result in deviation from the recommended imaging guidelines based on mechanism of injury and presenting symptoms. Low compliance with trauma imaging guidelines in pregnant patients has been reported in some centers.[22]

That being said, there is a consensus among many of the major trauma associations in the United States as well as the propensity of literature published in medical journals advocating to not withhold imaging with ionizing radiation from the pregnant trauma patient if indicated clinically. The Eastern Association for the Surgery of Trauma's most recently published guidelines for the diagnosis and management of injury in the pregnant patient clearly state this in their recommendations.[1] It is also emphasized in the current Advanced Trauma Life Support Curriculum developed by the American College of Surgeons as well as by Mattox and colleagues[11] in their textbook *Trauma*.

There have been no reported adverse fetal outcomes with regard to less than 5 rad of exposure and all common trauma imaging falls well below this threshold. The estimated fetal dose per computed tomography (CT) examination is as follows: CT head less than 0.05 rad, chest CT less than 0.1 rad, and abdomen and pelvis CT less than 2.6 rad.[1] While obtaining this imaging it is important to shield the uterus from excess radiation whenever possible.

When CT imaging of the abdomen and pelvis is obtained in the pregnant trauma patient, it may also prove helpful in evaluation for the diagnosis of placental abruption. Although this is traditionally diagnosed by ultrasonography or fetal distress noted on heart rate monitors, retrospective data have shown an 86% sensitivity, a 98% specificity, and a 96% overall accuracy of CT imaging in identifying the diagnosis of placental abruption.[23]

OUTCOMES

Data extracted from the National Trauma Data Bank revealed that pregnant women, when compared with nonpregnant women of the same age group who have similar injuries, are found to have a lesser mortality rate.[24] The physiologic reason for this is not fully understood; however, it has been reproduced in other retrospective reviews. It is counterintuitive, because we know that even minor traumatic injuries are often associated with increased fetal and maternal morbidity.

Data extracted from the Tennessee State Fetal Birth and Death Data System were reviewed for pregnant patients who were treated and discharged directly from the emergency room after what was defined as minor injury. In this group, minor injury during the first and second trimester was associated with increased risk for fetal demise, low birth rate, and prematurity.[25] Another group identified that minor traumatic injuries were associated with an increased risk for preterm labor. They went on to identify an increased risk for preterm labor, placental abruption, and uterine rupture, as well as maternal death in major traumatic injuries.[26]

The complications that affect the pregnant trauma patient are not always immediate and it is imperative that these patients be followed more closely through the remainder of their pregnancy. An Injury Severity Score of greater than 5 or the need for laparotomy during hospitalization have both been identified as independent predictors of long-term adverse pregnancy outcomes, including preterm labor, placental abruption, and perinatal morbidity.[27]

PERIMORTEM CESAREAN SECTION

The American College of Obstetrics and Gynecology advocates for perimortem cesarean section of the pregnant patient in extremis. This procedure is recommended in viable fetuses of at least 25 weeks gestation, reasonably expected to survive outside of the uterus. This procedure should be performed within 5 to 10 minutes of maternal cardiac arrest for acceptable outcomes. These recommendations are based more significantly on expert opinion and experience because there are limited data on this subject.

In 1 group of pregnant blunt trauma victims, 91 perimortem cesarean deliveries were performed and there was a reported fetal survival rate of 81% as well as a 34% maternal survival rate.[28] This is representative of the number most frequently quoted in the literature of a fetal survival rate of 70% if the perimortem cesarean is performed within 5 minutes of maternal death. Another study retrospectively reviewed 32 patients who underwent emergency cesarean section from 9 level 1 trauma centers in the United States. Thirty-three fetuses were delivered, 13 of which had no fetal heart tones before delivery and did not survive. Of the 20 (potential survivors) with fetal heart tones before delivery and an estimated gestational age of 26 weeks or greater, 75% survived. This group went on to recommend that infant viability in pregnant trauma patients in extremis is determined by the presence of fetal heart tones and estimated gestational age.[29]

An even more ethically controversial subject exists in the setting of the brain-dead pregnant trauma patient. The literature on this topic is sparse; however, the incidence of these cases is increasing as practices in critical care and resuscitation become more advanced. We have become more knowledgeable and equipped to maintain adequate perfusion in the setting of brain death and we often do this for organ donation, but to what extent in pregnancy? A systematic review article was published that summarized the case reports in the literature regarding the management of brain-dead pregnant mothers. Thirty cases were identified and the mean gestational age at the time of brain death was 22 weeks. The mean gestational age at the time of delivery was 29.5 weeks and 12 viable infants were born. There was minimal long-term follow-up, but all of the 12 survived the neonatal period.[30] This remains an infrequent occurrence that requires the input of many individuals, including the patient's family, the physicians caring for the patient, and an ethics team. It should continue to be handled on a case-by-case basis at this time.

REFERENCES

1. Barraco RD, Chiu WC, Clancy TV, et al. Practice management guidelines for the diagnosis and management of injury in the pregnant patient: the EAST Practice Management Guidelines Work Group. J Trauma 2010;69(1):211–4.
2. Mendez-Figueroa H, Dahlke JD, Vrees RA, et al. Trauma in pregnancy: an updated systematic review. Am J Obstet Gynecol 2013;209(1):1–10.
3. Fildes J, Reed L, Jones N, et al. Trauma: the leading cause of maternal death. J Trauma 1992;32(5):643–5.
4. Petrone P, Talving P, Browder T, et al. Abdominal injuries in pregnancy: a 155-month study at two level 1 trauma centers. Injury 2011;42(1):47–9.
5. Creanga AA, Berg CJ, Syverson C, et al. Pregnancy-related mortality in the United States, 2006-2010. Obstet Gynecol 2015;125(1):5–12.
6. McCrory JL, Chambers AJ, Daftary A, et al. Dynamic postural stability during advancing pregnancy. J Biomech 2010;43(12):2434–9.
7. Sanghavi M, Rutherford JD. Cardiovascular physiology of pregnancy. Circulation 2014;130(12):1003–8.
8. Hunter S, Robson SC. Adaptation of the maternal heart in pregnancy. Br Heart J 1992;68:540–3.
9. Rodger M, Sheppard D, Gandara E, et al. Haematological problems in obstetrics. Best Pract Res Clin Obstet Gynaecol 2015;29(5):671–84.
10. Hegewald MJ, Crapo RO. Respiratory physiology in pregnancy. Clin Chest Med 2011;32(1):1–12.
11. Mattox KL, Moore EE, Feliciano DV. Trauma. 7th edition. China: McGraw-Hill Companies, Inc; 2013.
12. Brown MA, Sirlin CB, Farahmand N, et al. Screening sonography in pregnant patients with blunt abdominal trauma. J Ultrasound Med 2005;24(2):175–81.

13. Williams J, Mozurkewich E, Chilimigras J, et al. Critical care in obstetrics: pregnancy-specific conditions. Best Pract Res Clin Obstet Gynaecol 2008; 22(5):825–46.
14. Tinker SC, Reefhuis J, Dellinger AM, et al. National birth defects prevention study. epidemiology of maternal injuries during pregnancy in a population-based study, 1997-2005. J Womens Health (Larchmt) 2010;19(12):2211–8.
15. Ikossi DG, Lazar AA, Morabito D, et al. Profile of mothers at risk: an analysis of injury and pregnancy loss in 1,195 trauma patients. J Am Coll Surg 2005; 200(1):49–56.
16. Weiss HB, Songer TJ, Fabio A. Fetal deaths related to maternal injury. JAMA 2001;286(15):1863–8.
17. Klinich KD, Flannagan CA, Rubb JD, et al. Fetal outcome in motor-vehicle crashes: effects of crash characteristics and maternal restraint. Am J Obstet Gynecol 2008;198(4):450.e1–9.
18. Motozawa Y, Hitosugi M, Abe T, et al. Effects of seat belts worn by pregnant drivers during low-impact collisions. Am J Obstet Gynecol 2010;203(1):62.e1–8.
19. Luley T, Fitzpatrick CB, Grotegut CA, et al. Perinatal implications of motor vehicle accident trauma during pregnancy: identifying populations at risk. Am J Obstet Gynecol 2013;208(6):466.e1–5.
20. Brookfield KF, Gonzalez-Quintero VH, Davis JS, et al. Maternal death in the emergency department from trauma. Arch Gynecol Obstet 2013;288(3):507–12.
21. Wiencrot A, Nannini A, Manning SE, et al. Neonatal outcomes and mental illness, substance abuse, and intentional injury during pregnancy. Matern Child Health J 2012;16(5):979–88.
22. Shakerian R, Thomson BN, Judson R, et al. Radiation fear: impact on compliance with trauma imaging guidelines in the pregnant patient. J Trauma Acute Care Surg 2015;78(1):88–93.
23. Manriguez M, Srinivas G, Bollepalli S, et al. Is computed tomography a reliable diagnostic modality in detecting placental injuries in the setting of acute trauma? Am J Obstet Gynecol 2010;202(6):611.e1–5.
24. John PR, Shiozawa A, Haut ER, et al. An assessment of the impact of pregnancy on trauma mortality. Surgery 2011;149(1):94–8.
25. Fischer PE, Zarzaur BL, Fabian TC, et al. Minor trauma is an unrecognized contributor to poor fetal outcomes: a population-based study of 78,552 pregnancies. J Trauma 2011;71(1):90–3.
26. Cheng HT, Want YC, Lo HC, et al. Trauma during pregnancy: a population-based analysis of maternal outcome. World J Surg 2012;36(12):2767–75.
27. Melamed N, Aviram A, Silver M, et al. Pregnancy course and outcome following blunt trauma. J Matern Fetal Neonatal Med 2012;25(9):1612–7.
28. Chibber R, Al-Harmi J, Fouda M, et al. Motor-vehicle injury in pregnancy and subsequent feto-maternal outcomes: of grave concern. J Matern Fetal Neonatal Med 2015;28(4):399–402.
29. Morris JA Jr, Rosenbower TJ, Jurkovich GJ, et al. Infant survival after cesarean section for trauma. Ann Surg 1996;223(5):481–8.
30. Esmaeilzadeh M, Dictus C, Kayvanpour E, et al. One life ends, another begins: management of a brain-dead pregnant mother-a systematic review. BMC Med 2010;8:74.

Maternal Sepsis and Septic Shock

Ahmad Chebbo, MD[a], Susanna Tan, MD[a], Christelle Kassis, MD[a],
Leslie Tamura, DO[a,b], Richard W. Carlson, MD, PhD[a,c,d],*

KEYWORDS

• Pregnancy • Sepsis • Severe sepsis • Septic shock

KEY POINTS

• Sepsis and septic shock are leading causes of intensive care unit admission as well as maternal and fetal morbidity and mortality.
• Early identification and management can be facilitated by various scoring systems.
• Physiologic changes of pregnancy and fetal oxygenation must be considered during resuscitation and management.
• The sites of infection as well as the organisms responsible for sepsis evolve throughout pregnancy, delivery, and postnatal intervals.
• Although not specifically developed for the pregnant patient, the Surviving Sepsis guidelines provide a useful paradigm for management.

INCIDENCE AND MORTALITY

Sepsis is the leading cause of death in the intensive care unit (ICU) and a common cause of morbidity and mortality worldwide.[1,2] Sepsis is also recognized as one of the major factors accounting for admission of pregnant patients to the ICU and for maternal death. Multiple studies over the years have documented an increase in the awareness of the precipitating factors and risks for sepsis in this special population.[3–10] The causative organisms, timing, prophylactic methods, and preventive strategies have been reviewed. Factors associated with the progression from severe sepsis to septic shock have also been identified. For pregnant women, there is a rapid progression from initial recognition of sepsis via defining parameters to development of severe sepsis and shock. In

Disclosures: The authors have no conflicts to report.
[a] Department of Medicine, Maricopa Medical Center, 2601 East Roosevelt, Phoenix, AZ 85008, USA; [b] Department of Medicine, Advocate Lutheran General Hospital, 1775 Dempster Street, 6 South, Park Ridge, IL 60068, USA; [c] Department of Medicine, Colleges of Medicine, University of Arizona, Phoenix, AZ, USA; [d] Department of Medicine, Mayo Clinic, Scottsdale, AZ, USA
* Corresponding author. Department of Medicine, Maricopa Medical Center, 2601 East Roosevelt, Phoenix, AZ 85008.
E-mail address: richardw_carlson@dmgaz.org

this regard, the normal underlying physiologic changes during pregnancy can critically alter hemodynamic stability when overlapped with sepsis. In concert with the most recent Surviving Sepsis campaign,[11] emphasis remains on timely recognition of sepsis and early administration of fluids and antibiotics. Sepsis accounted for 10.7% of maternal deaths from 2003 to 2012 according to the World Health Organization systematic analysis on the global causes of maternal death.[12] Trends of maternal mortality worldwide have been falling, but in the most recent report from the Centre for Maternal and Child Enquiries Mission statement in the United Kingdom, sepsis secondary to genital infections has become the leading cause of death, particularly from group A streptococcus (GAS).[9] There was an increase in maternal deaths related to sepsis from 0.85 of 100,000 pregnant women in 2003 to 2005 to 1.13 of 100,000 in 2006 to 2008.[9] Similarly, in a review of 2 tertiary referral maternity hospitals in Dublin, Ireland from 2005 to 2012 that included more than 150,000 pregnant women, the sepsis rate was 1.81 per 1000 pregnant women, of which 17% of the episodes occurred antenatally, 36% occurred intrapartum, and 47% occurred postpartum.[10] In a retrospective review on 74 patients admitted to the ICU, the rates of systemic inflammatory response syndrome (SIRS), severe sepsis, and septic shock are 59%, 24%, and 3%, respectively.[13] In a prospective study of 298 obstetric patients admitted to a tertiary referral ICU in Brazil, 14.2% of the admissions were caused by sepsis.[14] This increase may be attributed to women becoming pregnant after age 35 and presenting with higher rates of comorbidities.[15] Sepsis led to a high perinatal mortality as well as preterm delivery.[10] In the United States, similar trends have been observed. The incidence of pregnancy-associated severe sepsis (PASS) has increased by 236% over the last decade according to a study on 4,060,201 pregnancy-associated hospitalizations and 1077 PASS hospitalizations from 2001 to 2010.[16] The Centers for Disease Control and Prevention's Pregnancy Mortality Surveillance System recorded an increase in the number of reported pregnancy-related deaths in the United States. The pregnancy-related mortality ratio was 17.8 deaths per 100,000 live births according to the data from 2011, and 14% of the deaths were attributed to infection or sepsis, which was among the top 3 leading causes of pregnancy-related deaths (**Fig. 1**). As stated earlier, sepsis is also a major cause for admission of pregnant women to the ICU, together with hemorrhage, abortion, and complications of hypertension.[17]

DEFINITION

The definitions of SIRS, sepsis, severe sepsis, and septic shock for the nonpregnant patient are delineated in **Table 1**. However, there is currently no standard definition for severe sepsis for pregnant and peripartum women. There are multiple physiologic changes that occur in an obstetric patient during the antepartum and postpartum periods, which can mask some of the objective findings required to identify SIRS. Also, the accepted SIRS definition to identify patients with sepsis may be flawed. A recent study used data from 172 ICUs in Australia and in New Zealand that reviewed 1,171,797 patients admitted from 2003 to 2011 and found that using the current SIRS definition failed to identify up to 15% of patients with similar infections, organ failure, and risk of death.[18]

Accordingly, investigators have attempted to define severe sepsis, particularly for the pregnant patient. Barton and Sibai[15] defined a different set of parameters for severe sepsis and septic shock among obstetric patients that included a heart rate greater than 110 beats/min and respiratory rate greater than 24 breaths/min.

In addition, SIRS criteria may overlap with normal hemodynamic and other parameters during pregnancy and the peripartum period.[19] Those investigators conducted a

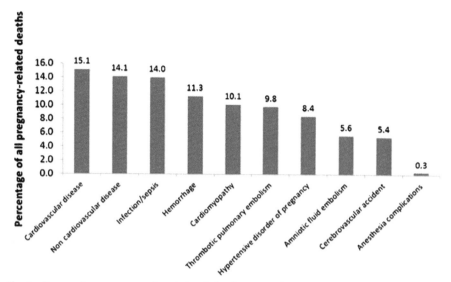

Fig. 1. Cause of pregnancy-related death in the United States: 2011. Note: The cause of death is unknown for 5.9% of all pregnancy-related deaths. (*From* CDC Pregnancy Mortality Surveillance System. Available at: http://www.cdc.gov/reproductivehealth/MaternalInfantHealth/PMSS.html.)

meta-analysis on 8834 healthy pregnant women, which revealed an overlap of 2 standard deviations above current SIRS criteria of heart rate, respiratory rate, and white blood cell count with the normal physiologic parameters during the second trimester, third trimester, and during labor, suggesting that other criteria may be needed to define maternal sepsis.[19]

PATHOPHYSIOLOGY OF SEPSIS

Sepsis is a complex, generalized, and overexpressed response by the host to an infection. On recognition of bacterial cell wall components and bacterial products such as endotoxins and exotoxins, the immune system initiates a cascade of events, including the release of pro-inflammatory mediators, release of cytokines by macrophages, recruitment of additional inflammatory cells, and activation of complement. These events lead to widespread cellular injury with ischemia, mitochondrial dysfunction, apoptosis, immunosuppression, multiple organ dysfunction, and death.[11] The response is modified by the patient's age, health status, and ability to compensate for the changes induced by the inflammatory response. Physiologic changes during pregnancy can contribute to an exaggerated septic response.

Immunologic Changes During Pregnancy

During pregnancy, there are immune response changes to protect the fetus from maternal inflammatory response. There is downregulation of cell-mediated immunity, with decreased T-cell activity secondary to a decrease in numbers or reduction in the CD4/CD8 ratio, with an intact or upregulated humoral response to balance this change. Because of this, there is a predisposition to certain infections, including *Listeria monocytogenes*, and more severe manifestations of some viral and fungal infections.[20]

Table 1
Definitions and parameters of systemic inflammatory response syndrome, severe sepsis, and septic shock

	Surviving Sepsis Campaign: International Guidelines for Management of Severe Sepsis and Septic Shock (Dellinger, 2012[11])	Clinical and Laboratory Findings of Severe Sepsis and Septic Shock (for Obstetric Patients) (Barton, 2012)
Infection	The invasion of normally sterile tissue by organisms	—
Bacteremia	Presence of viable bacteria in the blood	

SIRS	Two or more abnormalities in temperature, heart rate, respiration, or white blood count	General variables
		 • Fever (>38.3°C)
		 • Hypothermia (core temperature <36°C)
		 • Heart rate >90/min^{-1} or more than 2 SD above the normal value for age
		 • Tachypnea
		 • Altered mental status
		 • Significant edema or positive fluid balance (>20 mL/kg over 24 h)
		 • Hyperglycemia (plasma glucose >140 mg/dL or 7.7 mmol/L) in the absence of diabetes
		 Inflammatory variables
		 • Leukocytosis (WBC count >12,000 μL^{-1})
		 • Leukopenia (WBC count <4000 μL^{-1})
		 • Normal WBC count with >10% immature forms
		 • Plasma C-reactive protein more than 2 SD above the normal value
		 • Plasma procalcitonin more than 2 SD above the normal value
		 Hemodynamic variables
		 • Arterial hypotension (systolic blood pressure [SBP] <90 mm Hg, MAP <70 mm Hg, or an SBP decrease >40 mm Hg in adults or less than 2 SD below normal for age)
		 Organ dysfunction variables
		 • Arterial hypoxemia (PaO_2/FiO_2 <300)
		 • Acute oliguria (urine output <0.5 mL/kg/h for at least 2 h despite adequate fluid resuscitation)
		 • Creatinine increase >0.5 mg/dL or 44.2 μmol/L
		 • Coagulation abnormalities (INR >1.5 or aPTT >60 s)
		 • Ileus (absent bowel sounds)
		 • Thrombocytopenia (platelet count <100,000 μL^{-1})
		 • Hyperbilirubinemia (plasma total bilirubin > 4 mg/dL or 70 μmol/L)
		 Tissue perfusion variables
		 • Hyperlactatemia (>1 mmol/L)
		 • Decreased capillary refill or mottling
			Signs and symptoms of severe sepsis and septic shock
			 • Fever
			 • Temperature instability (>38°C or <36°C)
			 • Tachycardia (HR >100 bpm), tachypnea (RR >28/min)
			 • Diaphoresis
			 • Clammy/mottled skin
			 • Nausea/vomiting
			 • Hypotension/shock
			 • Oliguria
			 • Pain (location based on site of infection)
			 • Altered mental status (confusion, decreased alertness)
			 Laboratory findings in severe sepsis and septic shock
			 • Leukocytosis or leukopenia
			 • Hypoxemia
			 • Thrombocytopenia
			 • Metabolic acidosis
			   ○ Increased serum lactate
			   ○ Low pH
			   ○ Increased base deficit
			 • Elevated liver enzymes
			 • Disseminated intravascular coagulopathy
			 • Elevated serum creatinine

Sepsis	The presence (probable or documented) of infection together with systemic manifestations of infection	—
Severe sepsis	Sepsis plus sepsis-induced tissue hypoperfusion or organ dysfunction (any of the following thought to be due to the infection)	Sepsis-induced hypotension • Lactate above upper limits laboratory normal • Urine output <0.5 mL/kg/h for more than 2 h despite adequate fluid resuscitation • Acute lung injury with Pao_2/Fio_2 <250 in the absence of pneumonia as infection source • Acute lung injury with Pao_2/Fio_2 <200 in the presence of pneumonia as infection source • Creatinine >2.0 mg/dL (176.8 µmol/L) • Bilirubin >2 mg/dL (34.2 µmol/L) • Platelet count <100,000 µL • Coagulopathy (international normalized ratio >1.5)
Sepsis-induced hypotension	SBP <90 mm Hg or MAP <70 mm Hg or an SBP decrease >40 mm Hg or less than 2 SD below normal for age in the absence of other causes of hypotension	
Septic shock	Sepsis-induced hypotension despite adequate fluid resuscitation (infusion of 30 mL/kg of crystalloids)	
Multiple organ dysfunction syndrome	Progressive organ dysfunction in an acutely ill patient, such that hemostasis cannot be maintained without intervention	

Abbreviations: aPTT, activated partial thromboplastin time; HR, hazard ratio; INR, international normalized ratio; RR, relative risk; WBC, white blood cell count.
Adapted from Dellinger RP, Levy MM, Rhodes A, et al. Surviving Sepsis Campaign: international guidelines for management of severe sepsis and septic shock, 2012. Intensive Care Med 2013;39(2):165–228; and Barton JR, Sibai BM. Severe sepsis and septic shock in pregnancy. Obstet Gynecol 2012;120(3):689–706; with permission.

IDENTIFICATION/SCORING SYSTEMS

There are several scoring systems that have been used to identify patients at risk for sepsis and septic shock, including the Modified Early Warning Score (MEWS) and REMS score (Rapid Emergency Medicine Score). The MEWS has been used for emergency admissions to identity patients at risk for ICU admission and death. Lappen and colleagues[21] evaluated 913 chorioamnionitis patients using both SIRS and MEWS scores and found that neither can adequately identify patients at risk for sepsis, ICU transfer, or death. One of the reasons for failure of this scoring system to identify risk of morbidity in the obstetric population may be related to failure to take into account the normal physiologic changes seen in pregnancy, as described above (**Table 2**).

The Modified Early Obstetric Warning Score (MEOWS) is a tool designed specifically for the obstetric population, with a high sensitivity in predicting morbidity (89%) and reasonable specificity (79%) supporting its use for obstetric patients in predicting morbidity.[22] A validation study of the Confidential Enquiry into Maternal and Child Health Report (CEMACH) recommended modified early obstetric warning system (MEOWS). It is currently being used in the United Kingdom as recommended by the most recent CEMACH report,[9] but has not been widely used in North America.

The Sepsis in Obstetrics Score (S.O.S.) is another model that has been developed by Albright and colleagues to identify patients at high risk for admission to the ICU, specifically in an obstetric population group. A retrospective cohort study evaluated 850 women and compared S.O.S. with validated emergency department sepsis scoring systems, MEWS (cutoff of 5) and REMS (cutoff of 6), results of which are included in **Table 2**.

Risk Factors

Antepartum risk factors predisposing to perinatal sepsis include nonwhite ethnicity, obesity, lack of prenatal care, malnourishment, impaired glucose tolerance and diabetes mellitus, anemia, and impaired immunity. Patients with sickle cell disease or trait struggle to eliminate encapsulated bacteria due to poor splenic function. Immunosuppression due to HIV/AIDS compounded by opportunistic infections, such as tuberculosis, greatly increases the risk of severe postpartum infections.[4] History of group B streptococcal colonization or infection[7]; invasive procedures performed during pregnancy, such as sampling of chorionic villous, cervical cerclage, or amniocentesis[7,23,24]; black or minority ethnic origin, primiparous, pre-existing medical problems, febrile illness, and use of antibiotics in the 2 weeks before presentation also increased the odds of severe sepsis.[25]

Intrapartum risk factors include protracted active labor, especially in the nullipara, and prolonged rupture of membranes. More than 5 vaginal examinations increase

Table 2
Efficiency of scoring systems to predict sepsis

Scoring System	Sensitivity, %	Specificity, %	Positive Predictive Value, %	Negative Predictive Value, %
S.O.S.	88.9	99.2	16.7	99.9
REMS	77.8	93.3	11.1	99.7
MEWS	100	77.6	4.6	100

Data from Albright CM, Ali TN, Lopes V, et al. The Sepsis in Obstetrics Score: a model to identify risk of morbidity from sepsis in pregnancy. Am J Obstet Gynecol 2014;211:39.e1–8.

risk, together with perineal manipulation during the second stage of labor, as well as instrumentation at delivery.[13,23] Antibiotic prophylaxis for cesarean section is another risk. Finally, unscheduled cesarean section is the single most important risk factor for sepsis. Women who underwent cesarean section have a 5- to 20-fold greater risk for severe infections such as endometritis or wound infection compared with those who have a vaginal birth.[26]

Postpartum risk factors include retained placental fragments, cracked nipples, and operative delivery.[23] Operative vaginal delivery, prelabor cesarean section, and cesarean section after onset of labor also have increased odds of postpartum sepsis.[25] Risk factors associated with progression of sepsis include age greater than 25 years, high school education or less, public or no health insurance, and primary or repeat cesarean section.[4] Risk factors associated with progression to severe sepsis/septic shock include black, Asian, or Hispanic race, public or no health insurance, diabetes mellitus, chronic hypertension, delivery in a low-volume hospital (<1000 births/year), primiparity, multiple pregnancy, and postpartum hemorrhage.[4] In particular, multiple pregnancy and GAS as a causative organism have been associated with increased odds of progression to septic shock.[4,25]

Obesity is a significant emerging factor, and interestingly, the rates of both cesarean section and obesity have increased worldwide.[4] Poverty is still the most important determinant of maternal mortality from sepsis in developing countries. An avoidable risk factor in both high- and low-income countries is the failure to recognize severity of an infection by mothers, family members, birth attendants, and hospital staff (**Box 1**).

PREVENTION
Special Considerations: Maternal Cardiopulmonary Physiology and Fetal Oxygenation

An in-depth description of the dynamics of maternal physiology throughout pregnancy and the peripartum interval, as well as mechanisms of oxygen delivery to the fetus, is beyond the scope of this article, and the reader is referred to standard authorities on these topics. However, perturbations of these systems induced by severe sepsis can

---

Box 1
Techniques to prevent infections in pregnancy

1. Identify risks of contact with young children and individuals with recent pharyngitis

2. Perineal hygiene and hand washing

3. Prompt treatment of infections of other sites

4. Shower with antiseptic agent before surgery

5. Avoid smoking within 30 d of surgery

6. Glycemic control

7. Antimicrobial prophylaxis

8. Antenatal prophylaxis for premature rupture of membranes less than 37 weeks

9. Antibiotics for premature rupture of membranes greater than 37 weeks

10. Antibiotic prophylaxis for cesarean section

11. Broad spectrum antibiotics for obstetric and anal sphincter repair (3rd to 4th degree (Pelvic, laceration)

have profound effects on fetal and maternal viability. Accordingly, some aspects of maternal and fetal physiology that are likely to be affected during sepsis are summarized. **Fig. 2** depicts representative maternal and fetal physiologic issues.

As pregnancy progresses, there is a progressive increase in maternal blood volume of up to 150% by 32 weeks. Although red cell mass increases, expansion of plasma volume is greater, resulting in a modest decrease of hemoglobin, the "anemia of pregnancy."[27,28] Cardiac output and stroke volume also increase to 30% to 50% above prepregnancy values with a decrease in systemic vascular resistance.[29-35] Positional changes of the mother also modify venous return with obstruction of the vena cava by the gravid uterus.[36] Lateral decubitus or sitting posture improves venous return and hemodynamic parameters. During labor, cardiac output and arterial pressure increase, and each uterine contraction may be associated with an increase of 300 to 500 mL of venous return.[37,38] After delivery, there is an autotransfusion of up to 500 mL of blood from the uterus as well as removal of the gravid uterus as a source of vena caval obstruction. These changes may help offset blood loss during delivery. Fluid shifts from the extravascular fluid volume (ECF) to the vascular volume occur postpartum that may be augmented by intravenous fluids given during delivery. Serum proteins decline during pregnancy with a modest decrease of colloid osmotic pressure (COP) that may be further reduced by the ECF alterations cited above, hemorrhage, or administration of crystalloidal fluid. Further decreases of COP may be induced by alterations of vascular permeability by sepsis, increasing the risk of edema. Blood pressure returns to prepregnant values shortly after delivery, although increases in cardiac output and stroke volume may persist for a few weeks.[31,39-41] Although respiratory rate remains unchanged during pregnancy, there is an increase in tidal volume and minute ventilation. Maternal arterial blood gases reflect a modest respiratory alkalosis, with $Paco_2$ values of approximately 32 mm Hg induced in part by progesterone.[42-44] However, if $Paco_2$ values decrease to less than 30 mm Hg, there may be reductions of uterine blood flow. Renal blood flow is augmented during pregnancy, although during periods of stress, renal perfusion may be preferentially compromised with risk of acute renal injury.[29] In addition to the mild anemia of pregnancy cited earlier, there may be modest thrombocytopenia, which may be confused with or accentuated by sepsis.[29] Pregnancy is a procoagulant state, with up to a 4-fold increased risk of thromboses.[45] In addition, decreases in fibrinolytic activity during pregnancy may be further compromised by sepsis.

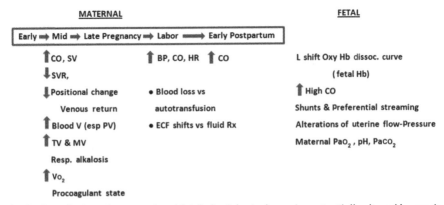

Fig. 2. Compilation of maternal and fetal physiologic dynamics potentially altered by sepsis. Blood V, blood volume; BP, arterial pressure; CO, cardiac output; MV, minute ventilation; PV, plasma volume; SV, stroke volume; TV, tidal volume; Vo_2, oxygen uptake–consumption.

Fetal transport and utilization of oxygen are complex processes and involve maternal pulmonary oxygenation and ventilation, uterine blood flow and pressure, maternal and fetal hemoglobin concentrations, as well as the oxygen tension gradient across the placenta. These changes are augmented by the left-shifted fetal oxyhemoglobin dissociation curve (ODC), maternal blood pH and $Paco_2$ umbilical blood flow, shunts and preferential streaming of blood within the fetus, together with the hyperdynamic fetal cardiovascular system.[46–48] Any or all of these components may be adversely affected during sepsis.

Maternal respiratory alkalosis favors the left-shifted ODC, affecting fetal oxygen loading as well as transport of CO_2 from fetus to the maternal circulation. Metabolic or respiratory acidosis of the mother may therefore adversely affect O_2 and CO_2 diffusion across the placenta. There must be a gradient of CO_2 tension from fetus to mother to eliminate fetal CO_2. Transient changes of these values are well usually well tolerated, but prolonged or severe disturbances of maternal pH, or $Paco_2$, may lead to fetal distress.[48–50] All of these factors are in turn affected by uterine blood flow and pressure. During pregnancy, maternal Pao_2 is normal, but fetal oxygen tensions are much lower with levels in the umbilical circulation of approximately 35 mm Hg and a corresponding saturation of 81%.[47,51] Hence, fetal oxygen delivery and utilization are dependent on a high fetal cardiac output, umbilical flow, shunts, and streaming of blood within the fetal circulation. Maternal hypoxemia can therefore have disastrous results on fetal oxygen delivery.

INFECTIONS DURING PREGNANCY AND THE PUERPERIUM: COMMON SITES THAT MAY LEAD TO SEPSIS AND ETIOLOGIC ORGANISMS

Infections of the genitalia or other sites can occur throughout pregnancy. The pregnant woman may develop similar infections as acquired during nonpregnant conditions, but there is a decrease in cell-mediated immune response in pregnancy, which may lead to greater predispositions for certain infections and a more severe response. There are also alterations of chest and abdominal cavities that may also lead to adverse outcomes for pneumonia.[52] In addition, the development of hydronephrosis as well as urinary reflux and high levels of progesterone is associated with a greater incidence of urinary infections. During labor and delivery, chorioamnionitis and endometritis may develop, particularly after extended labor, ruptured membranes, prior lower genital tract infections, and frequent vaginal examinations.[53] Therefore, most serious infections occurring during pregnancy affect the genitourinary systems. The evolution of etiologic agents during pregnancy, the intrapartum interval, and postnatal period is shown in **Table 3**.

PREGNANCY-ASSOCIATED GROUP A STREPTOCOCCAL INFECTIONS

GAS or *Streptococcus pyogenes* is a very virulent organism that can produce exotoxin, with extensive and rapidly developing tissue necrosis and maternal death.[54,55] The introduction of penicillin and antiseptic practice reduced the incidence of GAS,[56] but these infections re-emerged in 1980 with an annual incidence of 6 per 100,000 live births in the United States.[57] Compared with nonpregnant patients postpartum, women have a 20-fold increase in the incidence of GAS.[58] The increase may be related to breaches of mucosal barriers, alterations of vaginal pH, and decreased cellular immunity during pregnancy.

GAS presents with abdominal pain, fever, and tachycardia. Hypotension usually heralds the development of toxic shock syndrome and may be associated with up to 60% mortality, particularly if coupled with the development of renal failure.[56] Early diagnosis is thus crucial to prevent complications. Leukocytosis with marked

Table 3
Evolution of infectious organisms during pregnancy, intrapartum, and postnatal intervals

Organism	Antenatal	Intrapartum	Postnatal
E coli	55%	22%	42%
Group B streptococcus	4.2%	43%	9.2%
Anaerobes	8.5%	8%	8.5%
Staphylococcus	8.5%	5%	9.2%
Enterococcus	4.2%	5%	4.6%
G	0	2%	7.6%
Klebsiella	2%	2%	1.5%
H influenzae	6.4%	1%	0
Other	11.2%	11%	11.2%
Total, n	47	99	130

Data from Knowles SJ, O'Sullivan NP, Meenan AM. Maternal sepsis incidence, etiology and outcome for mother and fetus: a prospective study. BJOG 2015;122(5):663–71.

increases of immature white blood cells, together with fever and abdominal pain, should alert the clinician to consider GAS. Blood, urine, and endometrial aspiration should be performed, together with additional testing that may include computed tomographic (CT) imaging. Abdominal ultrasound may also be helpful. Aggressive and early resuscitation, antibiotics, and source control are keys to successful management. Penicillin G, together with Clindamycin, is the treatment of choice. Vancomycin may also be an alternative.[59] Duration of antibiotic therapy should be at least 14 days for patients with bacteremia or necrotizing fasciitis.

BACTERIAL PNEUMONIA

Similar microorganisms are generally recovered during pregnancy as for the nonpregnant patient. Although respiratory complications are frequently encountered, bacterial pneumonia occurs in only 0.1% to 0.2% of pregnancies.[60] Nevertheless, pneumonia is a major cause of maternal and fetal mortality[61] and is often misdiagnosed. It is also important to exclude and promptly treat viral causes of pneumonia.

An infectious agent can be isolated in 40% to 60% of patients with pneumonia.[61] Risk factors as well as signs and symptoms are similar to nonpregnant patients, although asthma is more common during pregnancy and may predispose to the development of pneumonia.[62]

Therapy for a healthy pregnant woman with uncomplicated community-acquired pneumonia is usually a macrolide. Doxycycline should be avoided and is contraindicated in pregnancy. Complicated or severe pneumonia should be managed with a macrolide plus a β-lactam.[63] Fluoroquinolones such as Levofloxacillin can also be considered a safe alternative[64] and are also effective against Legionella. Vancomycin can be added if Staphylococcal pneumoniae is suspected.

In addition to major complications such as septic shock and multiorgan failure, pneumonia during pregnancy is associated with a high incidence of preterm labor and delivery.[65]

PYELONEPHRITIS

Pyelonephritis is one of the more common severe infections during pregnancy and occurs in up to 2% of patients.[66] Because of compression of the gravid uterus, pyelonephritis predominately affects the right kidney. Etiologic organisms are usually similar to those in nonpregnant patients, with *Escherichia coli* a major pathogen. Other organisms, such as *Klebsiella* or *Proteus*, may also be recovered on culture, as well as more virulent organisms such as *Pseudomonas*. Patients who have underlying anatomic obstructive changes, instrumentation, or prior infections may also present with a variety of other organisms, although gram-positive and anaerobic organisms are seen less frequently in this population. For reasons that are not clear, acute respiratory distress syndrome occurs in up to 7% of pregnant patients with pyelonephritis.[20,67,68]

For patients with pyelonephritis who require hospitalization, therapy should include parenteral ceftriaxone.[69] Patients with severe or resistant infections should receive combination therapy that may include an aminoglycoside. Urine and blood cultures can guide selection for patients with uncommon or resistant organisms.

CHORIOAMNIONITIS

Chorioamnionitis (intra-amniotic infection) is a serious obstetric infection and is associated with increased risk of premature delivery and neonatal sepsis.[70] There is infection of the amniotic fluid, membranes, and placenta. Clinical infection complicates 1% of term pregnancies but may be more frequent with preterm delivery.[53,71] The route of infection is usually migration from the cervicovaginal area, with progression to the amnion, decidua, and amnionic fluid.[72] The infection is typically polymicrobial with a predominance of genital *Mycoplasma*, as well as *Streptococcus agalactiae* (*Streptococcus B*) and *E coli*.[73] Risk factors include prolonged labor, membrane rupture, digital vaginal examinations, presence of genital trace pathogens, young age, and alcohol use.[74] The patient presents with sepsis, uterine tenderness, and purulent discharge. Fever is present in almost all instances and is essential for diagnosis.[70] Bacteremia occurs in up to 10% of cases, especially with *E coli* and group B *Streptococcal* infection. Diagnosis can be confirmed with Gram stain and culture of amniotic fluid.

Empiric antibiotic coverage against anaerobes and aerobes should be initiated. One regimen includes Ampicillin with Gentamycin; Clindamycin can be added in patients undergoing cesarean section.[15,75] There is no benefit to continued oral antibiotics after parenteral therapy.[76]

Delivery will provide source control and prevent neonatal complications, but time to delivery does not appear to impact outcome.[71] Cesarean delivery is not indicated and should be reserved for the usual obstetric indications.

ENDOMETRITIS

In parallel with increases in the utilization of cesarean section, there has been a corresponding increase in the occurrence of endometritis, which remains a potentially life-threatening complication of abdominal delivery.[72] Postpartum endometritis is typically a polymicrobial infection that includes anaerobes in up to 40% of instances, together with a mixture of gram-positive and gram-negative facultative anaerobes.[77] Serious infections that are prone to lead to sepsis are caused by GAS, Staphylococci, and Clostridium species. Prolonged labor, cesarean section delivery, prolonged rupture of membranes, and multiple cervical examinations are risk factors.[78,79]

The patient presents with fever, tachycardia, and lower abdominal pain. Gram stain and culture of the uterine cavity is used to confirm the diagnosis and guide antibiotic therapy. Although ultrasound examination and CT scans can be used, the diagnosis is usually based on clinical features.

The choice of antibiotics should consider the polymicrobial nature of the infection: one regimen includes an aminoglycoside and clindamycin. Second- or third-generation cephalosporins, together with metronidazole, can also be used.[72,77] Duration of therapy should be guided by the clinical response; there is usually no need for extended oral therapy after response to parenteral antibiotics.[80]

MANAGEMENT

The guidelines developed by the Surviving Sepsis program can be used as a basis for the treatment of the pregnant woman with severe sepsis and septic shock, although the obstetric population was not specifically considered during the establishment of the guidelines and does not have provisions that consider the physiologic changes during pregnancy.[11] The clinician should also assess fetal viability as resuscitation and definitive management proceed.

Early recognition of sepsis is associated with improved mortality and outcome. However, in the young, otherwise healthy pregnant patient, delays in identification of sepsis may occur. Therefore, warning signs that may alert to severe sepsis include fever or hypothermia, tachycardia, tachypnea, diarrhea, vaginal discharge, leukopenia or leukocytosis, elevated lactate, metabolic acidosis, thrombocytopenia, or other manifestations of coagulopathy.[54] Utilization of a rapid response protocol that can detect early signs of sepsis and initiate additional evaluation with early and appropriate antibiotics and resuscitation has been linked to survival.[81,82]

Early goal-directed therapy (EGDT) aims to restore perfusion and tissue oxygenation by achieving physiologic targets during the early phases of resuscitation, including measurements of mean arterial pressure (MAP), central venous pressure (CVP), mixed venous oxygen saturation (SVO_2), and clearance of blood lactate.[83] EGDT has become a widely accepted standard of care in the management of severe sepsis and septic shock and has been applied to treatment of sepsis during pregnancy.[84] However, a recent study not involving pregnant patients did not observe a mortality benefit of EGDT resuscitation compared with usual care of patients with suspected sepsis in the emergency department.[85] In addition, some of the target values of the Rivers EGDT are different in pregnancy, such as cardiac output and SVO_2, which reflect a hyperdynamic state in pregnancy. In addition, by the third trimester, MAP is higher in the pregnant woman, together with a lower CVP and higher SVO_2.

Invasive hemodynamic monitoring using pulmonary artery flow-directed catheters has been used in pregnancy.[30] However, there are insufficient data to determine if invasive hemodynamic monitoring alters outcome during severe sepsis in pregnancy. If invasive hemodynamic monitoring is considered, the use of such devices and interpretation of hemodynamic parameters should be restricted to clinicians skilled in these techniques.[34] A variety of noninvasive techniques are now emerging to assess hemodynamic variables in the unstable patient.[29,31–34,39,86] Bedside ultrasound may be useful to guide fluid management, with assessment of inferior vena cava (IVC) size and collapse to various maneuvers, to estimate status of vascular volume and fluid responsiveness.[87] However, use of IVC changes to guide fluid resuscitation in pregnant patients has not been well studied, and positional effects as well as correlations with vascular volume may differ from the nonpregnant state.[36] A combination of invasive and noninvasive techniques is therefore recommended to achieve a functional approach to monitoring the unstable patient.[88] Once severe sepsis is suspected, restoration of perfusion should take priority by initiating antibiotics as well as fluid infusion. Using guidelines suggested above, an initial bolus of approximately 30 mL/kg should be given rapidly, using physiologic salt solution or lactated Ringer solution.[89] The choice of additional fluid remains controversial, but may include albumin. Synthetic colloidal solutions are not recommended.[90–92] Volume overload and pulmonary edema are potential hazards of vigorous volume resuscitation.

Vasoactive agents and additional blood products may be used if perfusion is not restored. Norepinephrine is typically the initial choice of a vasoactive agent, which may be augmented by epinephrine or vasopressin infusion.[93] Dopamine may be used for the patient with bradycardia. Dobutamine should be considered when an increase of cardiac output is a goal. Corticosteroids are currently recommended if the patient has refractory septic shock. The benefit of a random serum cortisol has been questioned.[94]

SUMMARY

Sepsis remains a major cause for admission of pregnant women to the ICU and is a leading cause of maternal morbidity and mortality. The Surviving Sepsis guideline continues to serve as a cornerstone for the diagnosis and management of sepsis, and many aspects of the management of severe sepsis are similar to that for the nonpregnant patient. However, both maternal and fetal morbidity and mortality are affected by the effectiveness of resuscitation and definitive therapy.

ACKNOWLEDGMENTS

The authors acknowledge the nursing and library staffs of Maricopa Medical Center, and Judy Hodgkins.

REFERENCES

1. Best M, Neuhauser D. Ignaz Semmelweis and the birth of infection control. Qual Saf Health Care 2004;13(3):233–4.
2. Semmelweis I. The etiology, concept, and prophylaxis of childbed fever (excerpts). Social Medicine 2008;3(1):4–12.
3. Acosta CD, Knight M. Sepsis and maternal mortality. Curr Opin Obstet Gynecol 2013;25(2):109–16.
4. Acosta CD, Knight M, Lee HC, et al. The continuum of maternal sepsis severity: incidence and risk factors in a population-based cohort study. PLoS One 2013; 8(7):e67175.
5. Bauer ME, Bateman BT, Bauer ST, et al. Maternal sepsis mortality and morbidity during hospitalization for delivery: temporal trends and independent associations for severe sepsis. Anesth Analg 2013;117(4):944–50.
6. Goff SL, Pekow PS, Avrunin J, et al. Patterns of obstetric infection rates in a large sample of US hospitals. Am J Obstet Gynecol 2013;208(6):456.e1–13.
7. Ford JM, Scholefield H. Sepsis in obstetrics: cause, prevention, and treatment. Curr Opin Anaesthesiol 2014;27(3):253–8.
8. Cordioli RL, Cordioli E, Negrini R, et al. Sepsis and pregnancy: do we know how to treat this situation? Rev Bras Ter Intensiva 2013;25(4):334–44.
9. Cantwell R, Clutton-Brock T, Cooper G, et al. Saving mothers' lives: reviewing maternal deaths to make motherhood safer: 2006-2008. the eighth report of the confidential enquiries into maternal deaths in the United Kingdom. BJOG 2011; 118(Suppl 1):1–203.
10. Knowles SJ, O'Sullivan NP, Meenan AM, et al. Maternal sepsis incidence, aetiology and outcome for mother and fetus: a prospective study. BJOG 2015; 122(5):663–71.

11. Dellinger RP, Levy MM, Rhodes A, et al. Surviving sepsis campaign: international guidelines for management of severe sepsis and septic shock: 2012. Crit Care Med 2013;41(2):580–637.

12. Say L, Chou D, Gemmill A, et al. Global causes of maternal death: a WHO systematic analysis. Lancet Glob Health 2014;2(6):e323–33.

13. Afessa B, Green B, Delke I, et al. Systemic inflammatory response syndrome, organ failure, and outcome in critically ill obstetric patients treated in an ICU. Chest 2001;120(4):1271–7.

14. Bandeira AR, Rezende CA, Reis ZS, et al. Epidemiologic profile, survival, and maternal prognosis factors among women at an obstetric intensive care unit. Int J Gynaecol Obstet 2014;124(1):63–6.

15. Barton JR, Sibai BM. Severe sepsis and septic shock in pregnancy. Obstet Gynecol 2012;120(3):689–706.

16. Oud L, Watkins P. Evolving trends in the epidemiology, resource utilization, and outcomes of pregnancy-associated severe sepsis: a population-based cohort study. J Clin Med Res 2015;7(6):400–16.

17. Ronsmans C, Graham WJ, Lancet Maternal Survival Series Steering Group. Maternal mortality: who, when, where, and why. Lancet 2006;368(9542):1189–200.

18. Kaukonen KM, Bailey M, Pilcher D, et al. Systemic inflammatory response syndrome criteria in defining severe sepsis. N Engl J Med 2015;372(17):1629–38.

19. Bauer ME, Bauer ST, Rajala B, et al. Maternal physiologic parameters in relationship to systemic inflammatory response syndrome criteria: a systematic review and meta-analysis. Obstet Gynecol 2014;124(3):535–41.

20. Lapinsky SE. Obstetric infections. Crit Care Clin 2013;29(3):509–20.

21. Lappen JR, Keene M, Lore M, et al. Existing models fail to predict sepsis in an obstetric population with intrauterine infection. Am J Obstet Gynecol 2010;203(6):573.e1–5.

22. Singh S, McGlennan A, England A, et al. A validation study of the CEMACH recommended modified early obstetric warning system (MEOWS). Anaesthesia 2012;67(1):12–8.

23. Burke C. Perinatal sepsis. J Perinat Neonatal Nurs 2009;23(1):42–51.

24. Simpson KR. Sepsis during pregnancy. J Obstet Gynecol Neonatal Nurs 1995;24(6):550–6.

25. Acosta CD, Kurinczuk JJ, Lucas DN, et al. Severe maternal sepsis in the UK, 2011-2012: a national case-control study. PLoS Med 2014;11(7):e1001672.

26. Smaill FM, Grivell RM. Antibiotic prophylaxis versus no prophylaxis for preventing infection after cesarean section. Cochrane Database Syst Rev 2014;(10):CD007482.

27. Clapp JF 3rd, Seaward BL, Sleamaker RH, et al. Maternal physiologic adaptations to early human pregnancy. Am J Obstet Gynecol 1988;159(6):1456–60.

28. Cavill I. Iron and erythropoiesis in normal subjects and in pregnancy. J Perinat Med 1995;23(1–2):47–50.

29. Carlin A, Alfirevic Z. Physiological changes of pregnancy and monitoring. Best Pract Res Clin Obstet Gynaecol 2008;22(5):801–23.

30. Clark SL, Cotton DB, Lee W, et al. Central hemodynamic assessment of normal term pregnancy. Am J Obstet Gynecol 1989;161(6 Pt 1):1439–42.

31. Gilson GJ, Samaan S, Crawford MH, et al. Changes in hemodynamics, ventricular remodeling, and ventricular contractility during normal pregnancy: a longitudinal study. Obstet Gynecol 1997;89(6):957–62.

32. Duvekot JJ, Cheriex EC, Pieters FA, et al. Early pregnancy changes in hemodynamics and volume homeostasis are consecutive adjustments triggered by a primary fall in systemic vascular tone. Am J Obstet Gynecol 1993;169(6):1382–92.

33. McNamara H, Barclay P, Sharma V. Accuracy and precision of the ultrasound cardiac output monitor (USCOM 1A) in pregnancy: comparison with three-dimensional transthoracic echocardiography. Br J Anaesth 2014;113(4):669–76.

34. Fujitani S, Baldisseri MR. Hemodynamic assessment in a pregnant and peripartum patient. Crit Care Med 2005;33(10 Suppl):S354–61.

35. Tan EK, Tan EL. Alterations in physiology and anatomy during pregnancy. Best Pract Res Clin Obstet Gynaecol 2013;27(6):791–802.

36. Ryo E, Unno N, Nagasaka T, et al. Changes in the size of maternal inferior vena cava during pregnancy. J Perinat Med 2004;32(4):327–31.

37. Hendricks CH, Quilligan EJ. Cardiac output during labor. Am J Obstet Gynecol 1956;71(5):953–72.

38. Robson SC, Dunlop W, Boys RJ, et al. Cardiac output during labour. Br Med J (Clin Res Ed) 1987;295(6607):1169–72.

39. Easterling TR, Benedetti TJ, Schmucker BC, et al. Maternal hemodynamics in normal and preeclamptic pregnancies: a longitudinal study. Obstet Gynecol 1990;76(6):1061–9.

40. Capeless EL, Clapp JF. When do cardiovascular parameters return to their preconception values? Am J Obstet Gynecol 1991;165(4 Pt 1):883–6.

41. Robson SC, Hunter S, Moore M, et al. Haemodynamic changes during the puerperium: a Doppler and M-mode echocardiographic study. Br J Obstet Gynaecol 1987;94(11):1028–39.

42. Bayliss DA, Millhorn DE. Central neural mechanisms of progesterone action: application to the respiratory system. J Appl Physiol (1985) 1992;73(2):393–404.

43. Spatling L, Fallenstein F, Huch A, et al. The variability of cardiopulmonary adaptation to pregnancy at rest and during exercise. Br J Obstet Gynaecol 1992; 99(Suppl 8):1–40.

44. Lapinsky SE, Kruczynski K, Slutsky AS. Critical care in the pregnant patient. Am J Respir Crit Care Med 1995;152(2):427–55.

45. Heit JA, Kobbervig CE, James AH, et al. Trends in the incidence of venous thromboembolism during pregnancy or postpartum: a 30-year population-based study. Ann Intern Med 2005;143(10):697–706.

46. Fineman JR, Clyman R. Fetal cardiovascular physiology. In: Creasy RK, Resnik R, Iams JD, et al, editors. Philadelphia: Elsevier; 2014. p. 146–54.

47. Meschia G. Placental respiratory gas exchange and fetal oxygenation. In: Creasy RK, Resnik R, Iams JD, et al, editors. Philadelphia: Elsevier; 2014. p. 163–74.

48. Bergmans MG, Stevens GH, Keunen H, et al. Transcutaneous and arterial carbon dioxide tension at various conditions of fetal stress in lambs. Gynecol Obstet Invest 1997;43(1):1–5.

49. Fraser D, Jensen D, Wolfe LA, et al. Fetal heart rate response to maternal hypocapnia and hypercapnia in late gestation. J Obstet Gynaecol Can 2008;30(4): 312–6.

50. Cook PT. The influence on foetal outcome of maternal carbon dioxide tension at caesarean section under general anaesthesia. Anaesth Intensive Care 1984; 12(4):296–302.

51. Minnich ME, Brown M, Clark RB, et al. Oxygen desaturation in women in labor. J Reprod Med 1990;35(7):693–6.

52. Goodrum LA. Pneumonia in pregnancy. Semin Perinatol 1997;21(4):276–83.

53. Duff P. Maternal and perinatal infection. In: Gabbe SG, editor. Obstetrics: Normal and Preterm Pregnancies. Philadelphia: Elsevier/Saunders; 2012. p. 1140–55.
54. Sriskandan S. Severe peripartum sepsis. J R Coll Physicians Edinb 2011;41(4): 339–46.
55. Norwitz E, Lee H. Septic shock. In: Belfort MA, Saade G, Foley MR, et al, editors. Critical Care Obstetrics. Hoboken (NJ): Wiley-Blackwell; 2010. p. 571–95.
56. Rimawi BH, Soper DE, Eschenbach DA. Group A streptococcal infections in obstetrics and gynecology. Clin Obstet Gynecol 2012;55(4):864–74.
57. Chuang I, Van Beneden C, Beall B, et al. Population-based surveillance for postpartum invasive group a streptococcus infections, 1995-2000. Clin Infect Dis 2002;35(6):665–70.
58. Deutscher M, Lewis M, Zell ER, et al. Incidence and severity of invasive Streptococcus pneumoniae, group A Streptococcus, and group B Streptococcus infections among pregnant and postpartum women. Clin Infect Dis 2011;53(2):114–23.
59. Stevens DL, Bisno AL, Chambers HF, et al. Practice guidelines for the diagnosis and management of skin and soft tissue infections: 2014 update by the Infectious Diseases Society of America. Clin Infect Dis 2014;59(2):e10–52.
60. Munn MB, Groome LJ, Atterbury JL, et al. Pneumonia as a complication of pregnancy. J Matern Fetal Med 1999;8(4):151–4.
61. Goodnight WH, Soper DE. Pneumonia in pregnancy. Crit Care Med 2005;33(10 Suppl):S390–7.
62. Yost NP, Bloom SL, Richey SD, et al. An appraisal of treatment guidelines for antepartum community-acquired pneumonia. Am J Obstet Gynecol 2000;183(1): 131–5.
63. Harrison BD, Farr BM, Connolly CK, et al. The hospital management of community-acquired pneumonia. Recommendations of the British Thoracic Society. J R Coll Physicians Lond 1987;21(4):267–9.
64. Cunha BA. Empiric therapy of community-acquired pneumonia: guidelines for the perplexed? Chest 2004;125(5):1913–9.
65. Banhidy F, Acs N, Puho EH, et al. Maternal acute respiratory infectious diseases during pregnancy and birth outcomes. Eur J Epidemiol 2008;23(1):29–35.
66. Duff P. Pyelonephritis in pregnancy. Clin Obstet Gynecol 1984;27(1):17–31.
67. Hill JB, Sheffield JS, McIntire DD, et al. Acute pyelonephritis in pregnancy. Obstet Gynecol 2005;105(1):18–23.
68. Cole DE, Taylor TL, McCullough DM, et al. Acute respiratory distress syndrome in pregnancy. Crit Care Med 2005;33(10 Suppl):S269–78.
69. Duff P. Antibiotic selection in obstetrics: making cost-effective choices. Clin Obstet Gynecol 2002;45(1):59–72.
70. Tita AT, Andrews WW. Diagnosis and management of clinical chorioamnionitis. Clin Perinatol 2010;37(2):339–54.
71. Gibbs RS, Duff P. Progress in pathogenesis and management of clinical intraamniotic infection. Am J Obstet Gynecol 1991;164(5 Pt 1):1317–26.
72. Casey BM, Cox SM. Chorioamnionitis and endometritis. Infect Dis Clin North Am 1997;11(1):203–22.
73. Galask RP, Varner MW, Petzold CR, et al. Bacterial attachment to the chorioamniotic membranes. Am J Obstet Gynecol 1984;148(7):915–28.
74. Soper DE, Mayhall CG, Dalton HP. Risk factors for intraamniotic infection: a prospective epidemiologic study. Am J Obstet Gynecol 1989;161(3):562–6 [discussion: 566–8].
75. Black LP, Hinson L, Duff P. Limited course of antibiotic treatment for chorioamnionitis. Obstet Gynecol 2012;119(6):1102–5.

76. Dinsmoor MJ, Newton ER, Gibbs RS. A randomized, double-blind, placebo-controlled trial of oral antibiotic therapy following intravenous antibiotic therapy for postpartum endometritis. Obstet Gynecol 1991;77(1):60–2.

77. Rosene K, Eschenbach DA, Tompkins LS, et al. Polymicrobial early postpartum endometritis with facultative and anaerobic bacteria, genital mycoplasmas, and Chlamydia trachomatis: treatment with piperacillin or cefoxitin. J Infect Dis 1986;153(6):1028–37.

78. D'Angelo LJ, Sokol RJ. Time-related peripartum determinants of postpartum morbidity. Obstet Gynecol 1980;55(3):319–23.

79. Diamond MP, Entman SS, Salyer SL, et al. Increased risk of endometritis and wound infection after cesarean section in insulin-dependent diabetic women. Am J Obstet Gynecol 1986;155(2):297–300.

80. French LM, Smaill FM. Antibiotic regimens for endometritis after delivery. Cochrane Database Syst Rev 2004;(4):CD001067.

81. Kumar A, Roberts D, Wood KE, et al. Duration of hypotension before initiation of effective antimicrobial therapy is the critical determinant of survival in human septic shock. Crit Care Med 2006;34(6):1589–96.

82. Kumar A, Ellis P, Arabi Y, et al. Initiation of inappropriate antimicrobial therapy results in a fivefold reduction of survival in human septic shock. Chest 2009;136(5): 1237–48.

83. Rivers E, Nguyen B, Havstad S, et al. Early goal-directed therapy in the treatment of severe sepsis and septic shock. N Engl J Med 2001;345(19):1368–77.

84. Guinn DA, Abel DE, Tomlinson MW. Early goal directed therapy for sepsis during pregnancy. Obstet Gynecol Clin North Am 2007;34(3):459–79, xi.

85. ProCESS Investigators, Yealy DM, Kellum JA, et al. A randomized trial of protocol-based care for early septic shock. N Engl J Med 2014;370(18):1683–93.

86. Burlingame J, Ohana P, Aaronoff M, et al. Noninvasive cardiac monitoring in pregnancy: impedance cardiography versus echocardiography. J Perinatol 2013; 33(9):675–80.

87. Cardenas-Garcia J, Mayo PH. Bedside ultrasonography for the intensivist. Crit Care Clin 2015;31(1):43–66.

88. Pinsky MR. Functional hemodynamic monitoring. Crit Care Clin 2015;31(1): 89–111.

89. Myburgh JA, Mythen MG. Resuscitation fluids. N Engl J Med 2013;369(13): 1243–51.

90. Delaney AP, Dan A, McCaffrey J, et al. The role of albumin as a resuscitation fluid for patients with sepsis: a systematic review and meta-analysis. Crit Care Med 2011;39(2):386–91.

91. Myburgh JA, Finfer S, Bellomo R, et al. Hydroxyethyl starch or saline for fluid resuscitation in intensive care. N Engl J Med 2012;367(20):1901–11.

92. Perner A, Haase N, Guttormsen AB, et al. Hydroxyethyl starch 130/0.42 versus Ringer's acetate in severe sepsis. N Engl J Med 2012;367(2):124–34.

93. Robbins KS, Martin SR, Wilson WC. Intensive care considerations for the critically ill parturient. In: Creasy RK, Resnik R, Iams JD, et al, editors. Maternal-Fetal Medicine: Principles and Practice. Boston: Elsevier Saunders; 2014. p. 1182–211.

94. Sprung CL, Annane D, Keh D, et al. Hydrocortisone therapy for patients with septic shock. N Engl J Med 2008;358(2):111–24.

Ethical Issues in Maternal–Fetal Care Emergencies

Nyima Ali, MD[a],*, Dean V. Coonrod, MD, MPH[a,b], Thomas R. McCormick, DMin[c]

KEYWORDS

- Maternal ethics • Emergency ethics • Maternal emergencies • Domestic violence
- Ethical emergencies

KEY POINTS

- Even in situations of questionable maternal decision making, a physician should begin with the framework that the pregnant woman and the fetus are interconnected and interdependent.
- The American Congress of Obstetrics and Gynecologists (ACOG) Committee on Ethics has stated opposition to the criminal prosecution of pregnant women whose activities seem to cause fetal harm.
- Communication by the primary physician with all members of the team and family cannot be stressed enough; appropriate informed consent is vital to resolution of managing a brain-dead pregnant patient.
- It is most therapeutic when a woman is empowered to independently disclose cases of domestic violence.
- In cases of domestic violence, fetal rights have not been so compelling to bypass a women's autonomous decision to not intervene on behalf of the fetus.

INTRODUCTION

Ethical issues that arise in the care of pregnant women are challenging to physicians, especially in critical care situations. By familiarizing themselves with the concepts of medical ethics in obstetrics, physicians will become more capable of approaching complex ethical situations with a clear and structured framework. This framework allows physicians to balance principles, human virtues, care and holistic perspectives, and concern for community, and to establish case precedents. This balance

Disclosures: None.
[a] Department of Obstetrics and Gynecology, Maricopa Integrated Health System, District Medical Group, 2601 E Roosevelt, Phoenix, AZ 85008, USA; [b] Department of Obstetrics and Gynecology, University of Arizona College of Medicine, 550 E Van Buren Street, Phoenix, AZ 85004, USA; [c] Department Bioethics and Humanities, University of Washington, Seattle, WA 98195-7120, USA
* Corresponding author.
E-mail address: Nyima_Ali@dmgaz.org

enhances their ability to make clinical decisions, grounded in sound ethics, which are justifiable to a diverse group of constituents. Often, more than 1 course of action is justifiable morally. At times, however, no course of action may seem acceptable; each course of action may result in significant harms or compromise important principles or values.[1] The time frame for considering and choosing a course of action is also often short. Despite these demands, the clinician is obliged to apply the same critical thinking faculties that would be applied to issues of medical evidence, select one of the available options, and justify this decision through communication of his or her ethical reasons.[1] The goals of this article are to review 3 specific situations in emergency maternal care ethics, identify issues requiring clarification/further understanding, and help to construct a framework in which to make an ethically sound decision.

LIFE OF THE FETUS VERSUS LIFE OF THE MOTHER AND SITUATIONS OF QUESTIONABLE MATERNAL DECISION MAKING

Practitioners who care for pregnant women face difficult dilemmas when their patients reject medical recommendations. This dilemma is particularly more complex when the rejection of medical recommendations clearly causes significant fetal harm (eg, when a pregnant woman uses illegal drugs or abuses alcohol). As a general precedent, most ethicists and the American Congress of Obstetrics and Gynecologists (ACOG) agree that a pregnant woman's informed refusal of medical intervention should take precedence, as long as she has the ability to make medical decisions.[1] This discussion presents a review of the general ethical considerations applicable to pregnant women who do not follow the advice of their physicians or do not seem to make decisions in the best interest of their fetuses.

One framework treats the woman and her fetus as separable and independent. Although this separation is meant to simplify and add clarity to complex obstetrics issues, many writers have noted that such frameworks tend to distort, rather than illuminate, ethical and policy debates.[1,2] This distortion occurs because the view of mother and fetus as separate entities overlooks the shared interests of the pregnant woman and fetus. When viewing the maternal–fetal relationship as divergent, and by extension possibly adversarial, one ignores that the interests of the pregnant woman and fetus actually converge, creating a unique and sensitive interdependency between the mother and her future child.[3]

A more appropriate framework recognizes that the pregnant woman and the fetus are interconnected and interdependent.[1,3] For example, a fetal intervention must be performed through the pregnant woman. Thus, the fetus depends on the mother for necessary medical care. Another example highlights the moral relationship between the pregnant woman and the fetus. When abstracting the fetus from the pregnant woman, the woman herself may suffer from a moral injury. The woman in this case is a patient, a person, and a bearer of moral rights.[2–4] Extending these examples further, recognizing the role of the pregnant woman exemplifies a fundamental moral principle: persons are never treated solely as means to an end, but as ends in themselves.

Another framework within medical ethics calls for health care professionals to respect their patients' autonomous decisions, which are highlighted by following the requirement for informed consent before undertaking a medical intervention.[2,3] Pregnancy is not an item that removes or limits informed consent. As noted, fetal interventions require performing a procedure on the body of the pregnant mother. This necessitates taking the woman's informed consent.[2] Regarding informed consent, in January 2004, the ACOG Committee on Ethics published a bulletin in which the following points are noted:

- "Requiring informed consent is an expression of respect for the patient as a person; it particularly respects a patient's moral right to bodily integrity, to self-determination regarding sexuality and reproductive capacities, and to the support of the patient's freedom within caring relationships."
- "The ethical requirement for informed consent need not conflict with physicians' overall ethical obligation to a principle of beneficence; that is, every effort should be made to incorporate a commitment to informed consent within a commitment to provide medical benefit to patients and thus respect them as whole and embodied persons."

When obtaining informed consent, the physician must both give clear, comprehensive advice and also offer assistance to help pregnant women who seek help in following this advice (eg, answering their questions, suggesting support resources).[5] As in any medical situation, the pregnant woman may ignore this advice, which is within her rights as an autonomous being.[6,7] The issues associated with informed refusal of care by pregnant women are addressed in the January 2004 opinion "Patient Choice in the Maternal–Fetal Relationship."[3] This opinion states that in cases of maternal refusal of treatment for the sake of the fetus, "court-ordered intervention against the wishes of a pregnant woman is rarely if ever acceptable."

In their committee opinion on maternal decision making,[1] ACOG has noted the following objections to punitive and coercive legal approaches to maternal decision making. These approaches:

1. Fail to recognize that pregnant women are entitled to informed consent and bodily integrity;
2. Fail to recognize that medical knowledge and predictions of outcomes in obstetrics have limitations;
3. Treat addiction and psychiatric illness as if they were moral failings;
4. Threaten to dissuade women from prenatal care;
5. Unjustly single out the most vulnerable women; and
6. Create the potential for criminalization of otherwise legal maternal behavior.

Based on these 6 considerations, the ACOG Committee on Ethics has stated a clear opposition to the criminal prosecution of pregnant women whose activities seem to cause fetal harm.[1] Instead, the ACOG Committee on Ethics makes recommends the following:

- In caring for pregnant women, practitioners should recognize that in the majority of cases, the interests of the pregnant woman and her fetus converge rather than diverge. Promoting pregnant women's health through advocacy of healthy behavior, referral for substance abuse treatment and mental health services when necessary, and maintenance of a good physician–patient relationship is always in the best interest of both the woman and her fetus.
- Pregnant women's autonomous decisions should be respected. Concerns about the impact of maternal decisions on fetal well-being should be discussed in the context of medical evidence and understood within the context of each woman's broad social network, cultural beliefs, and values.
- Pregnant women should not be punished for adverse perinatal outcomes. The relationship between maternal behavior and perinatal outcome is not fully understood, and punitive approaches threaten to dissuade pregnant women from

seeking health care and ultimately undermine the health of pregnant women and their fetuses.

- Policy makers, legislators, and physicians should work together to find constructive and evidence-based ways to address the needs of women with alcohol and other substance abuse problems.[4]

WITHDRAWAL OF CARE IN A BRAIN-DEAD PREGNANT PATIENT

Brain injury in a pregnant woman most commonly results from either trauma or intracranial abnormalities, such as an aneurysm that ruptures, causing hemorrhage or stroke. These casualties may lead to maternal brain death.[8] Maternal somatic support after brain death occurs when a brain-dead patient is pregnant and her body is kept alive to deliver a fetus. It is a very rare occurrence. In a US study of 252 brain dead patients from the mid 1990s, only 5 cases (2.8%) involved pregnant women between 15 and 45 years of age.[9]

Terminology

Patients in a persistent vegetative state are alive but also have severely impaired consciousness, although their eyes may open spontaneously.[9,10] A vegetative state means "permanent and total loss of forebrain function," which needs further investigation and monitoring.[10] In the US legal system, courts may require petitions before termination of life support that demonstrate that any recovery of cognitive functions above a vegetative state is assessed as impossible by authoritative medical opinion. Brain death means the "death of the brainstem," which can be clinically diagnosed by standard diagnostic procedures such as an electroencephalogram. People in comas have presence of brainstem responses, spontaneous breathing, or nonpurposeful motor responses but comas can lead to brain death, or recovery or a persistent vegetative state depending on the extent of the injury.[9,10]

Brain death implies absolute and incontrovertible cessation of total brain function, including brainstem function. Supportive interventions are mandatory if somatic functions are to be preserved, in particular ventilation and circulation.[8,9] A pregnant woman who has been diagnosed as brain dead is considered dead, and somatic support is justified only to design appropriate strategies for the sake of the fetus.

Pregnancy adds considerable complexity to maintenance of life support. Maternal supportive care may last for many weeks to achieve fetal viability outside of the uterus, far longer than what is required for supportive care for organ donation. Once continuation of pregnancy has been decided after maternal brain death, systemic vital functions must be supported actively to maintain a maternal milieu as close as possible to the physiologic state of pregnancy.[8]

The decision about whether attempts to maintain pregnancy are likely to be successful depends first on the gestational age of the fetus. For brain death in early pregnancy, supportive care may lead to the birth of a desperately premature neonate. However, starting at 12 to 14 weeks of gestation, fetal survival has been successfully prolonged for 15 weeks, bringing the fetus beyond the threshold of viability (approximately 23 weeks after the last menstrual period).[8] Questions regarding maintaining pregnancy must be answered in consultation with a spouse, next of kin, or designated decision maker. This discussion may not always be possible given the urgency, rarity, and gravity of the situation. In the absence of any expressed wish of the woman, her preference for the future of her fetus, to be kept alive or not, must be discussed. A substitute decision maker must be identified by the practitioner and must act in the interests of the woman's respectful treatment. Transfer to a higher level maternity care hospital with appropriate facilities, counseling services, and coordination of care is of utmost importance to achieve an optimal outcome in these situations. The primary physicians in this circumstance may play several roles to ensure all facets of care and decision making are being met.

Another important issue to consider is the financial burden associated with life support. The cost of maintaining a brain-dead pregnant woman to deliver a child is very expensive and the availability and just allocation of human and material resources is a matter of tremendous concern. Public and private health insurance plans do not usually cover services after death is determined. After maternal wishes and best interests are considered, the best interests of the fetus must also be considered, even where the fetus is in law not yet a person.[11] Among the issues to be considered are the viability of the fetus and its probable health status before and after birth. All reasonable efforts should be made to promote the birth of an adequately mature, brain-intact neonate.[8]

An analysis of the various factors involved in ethical decisions can aid attempts to resolve difficult cases. In addition, the involvement of individuals with a variety of backgrounds and perspectives can be useful in addressing ethical questions. Informal or formal consultation with those from related services or with a hospital ethics committee can help to ensure that all stakeholders, viewpoints, and options are considered as a decision is made.

Given the rarity of the situation, communication by the primary physician with all members of the team (including but not limited to obstetric, neonatal, intensive care, trauma/surgery, maternal–fetal medicine, hospital ethics, spiritual, and financial representatives) and family cannot be stressed enough. Adequate communication with discussion involving appropriate informed consent is vital to an optimal resolution of such a case.

DOMESTIC VIOLENCE AND THE PREGNANT PATIENT

Similar to issues arising from alcohol and substance use are issues of a pregnant woman living with domestic violence. Should a provider be obligated to report such abuse to justice authorities, even against the will of the patient? In some jurisdictions, domestic violence is reportable just as child abuse requires mandatory reporting. Arguments against this include loss of autonomy of a competent adult, that mandatory reporting represents a paternalistic approach, and responding to the domestic violence victim in a disempowering manner.[12] This tactic is contradictory to a therapeutic approach of allowing a victim to be empowered to act against the power and control that is central to the perpetrator's motivation to abuse. Furthermore, it has been argued that mandatory reporting would be a barrier to disclosure.[12] One suggested way to allow for empowerment when making a query about domestic violence in the setting of mandatory reporting is to inform the patient of a requirement to report, thus allowing the victim to make an informed and possibly empowering decision to disclose. In other jurisdictions, material injury and assault with a deadly weapon require reporting.[12] Given that domestic violence in pregnancy is deemed a risk factor for lethality,[13,14] does identified violence in pregnancy require a report? Most argue that a risk factor does not carry the weight of an identified injury or use of a deadly weapon.

As noted, fetal rights have not been generally so compelling to bypass a women's autonomous decision to not intervene on behalf of the fetus. This is rooted in the lack of "personhood" granted to the fetus. This reaches certain poignancy when considering a lethal act of domestic violence in which the victim and the unborn fetus expire.

In the past, the death of the fetus was not considered a separate crime but merely a detail of a crime. After the murder of a wife and the death of an unborn fetus in a high-profile crime,[15] the Unborn Victims of Violence Act of 2004[16] was passed by the US Congress and signed into law. This act considers the death of the fetus a separate crime because it carries the presumption that as a potential child it was destined to have a life and thus its injury or death in the course of a crime is a punishable offense. This law excludes abortion, for which the woman consents, as an offense and excludes those providing medical treatment from being prosecuted. The authors of this article are not aware of prosecutions of women for injury to their fetus for continued substance use, refusing medical care, or even more perversely remaining in a domestic violence situation. As a result, most experts recommend an approach of screening and providing options to a woman who discloses domestic abuse in a pregnancy.[17]

SUMMARY

Ethical issues that arise in the care of pregnant women are challenging to physicians, especially in critical care situations. This review discusses ethical approaches regarding 3 specific scenarios: (1) the life of the fetus versus the life of the mother and situations of questionable maternal decision making, (2) withdrawal of care in a brain-dead pregnant patient, and (3) domestic violence and the pregnant patient. When presented to the provider in the emergent setting, more than 1 course of action is morally justifiable and, sometimes, no course of action may seem acceptable; each course of action may result in significant harms or compromise important principles or values.[1] Even in situations of questionable maternal decision making, a physician should begin with the framework that the pregnant woman and the fetus are interconnected and interdependent. Communication and coordination of care by the primary physician with all members of the team (including but not limited to obstetric, neonatal, intensive care, trauma/surgery, maternal fetal medicine, hospital ethics, spiritual, and financial representatives) and family is vital to achieving an optimal outcome. By using evidence-based medical principles with sound ethical rationale and effective communication tools, the obstetrician and intensivist can be better prepared for such emergent situations.

REFERENCES

1. Maternal decision making, ethics and the law. American College of Obstetricians and Gynecologists; 2005. Committee on Ethics. Number 321. Available at: http://www.acog.org/Resources-And-Publications/Committee-Opinions/Committee-on-Ethics/Informed-Consent.
2. Informed consent. In: American College of Obstetricians and Gynecologists, editor. Ethics in obstetrics and gynecology. 2nd edition. Washington, DC: American College of Obstetricians and Gynecologists; 2004. p. 9–17.
3. Patient choice in the maternal–fetal relationship. In: American College of Obstetricians and Gynecologists, editor. Ethics in obstetrics and gynecology. 2nd edition. Washington, DC: American College of Obstetricians and Gynecologists; 2004. p. 34–6.
4. ACOG Committee on Ethics. ACOG Committee Opinion. Number 294, May 2004. At-risk drinking and illicit drug use: ethical issues in obstetric and gynecologic practice. Obstet Gynecol 2004;103:1021–31.

5. American College of Obstetrics and Gynecology. ACOG Committee Opinion No. 390. Ethical decision making in obstetrics and gynecology. Obstet Gynecol 2007; 110:1479–87.
6. ACOG Committee on Ethics. ACOG Committee Opinion No. 358. Professional responsibilities in obstetric–gynecologic education. Obstet Gynecol 2007;109: 239–42.
7. President's Commission for the Study of Ethical Problems in Medicine and Biomedical and Behavioral Research. Making health care decisions: the ethical and legal implications of informed consent in the patient-practitioner relationship. Washington, DC: U.S. Government Printing Office; 1982.
8. Ethical issues in obstetrics and gynecology by the FIGO Committee for the Study of Ethical Aspects of Human Reproduction and Women's Health. 2012.
9. Suddaby EC, Schaeffer MJ, Brigham LE, et al. Analysis of organ donors in the peripartum period. J Transpl Coord 1998;8(1):35–9.
10. Young B, Blume W, Lynch A. Brain death and the persistent vegetative state: similarities and contrasts. Can J Neurol Sci 1989;16(4):388–93.
11. American College of Obstetricians and Gynecologists Committee on Ethics. Committee Opinion No. 480. Empathy in women's health care. Obstet Gynecol 2011;117:756–61.
12. Hyman A, Chez RA. Mandatory reporting of domestic violence by health care providers: a misguided approach. Womens Health Issues 1995;5(4):208–13.
13. Campbell JC, Glass N, Sharps PW, et al. Intimate partner homicide: review and implications of research and policy. Trauma Violence Abuse 2007;8(3):246–69.
14. McFarlane J, Campbell JC, Sharps P, et al. Abuse during pregnancy and femicide: urgent implications for women's health. Obstet Gynecol 2002;100(1):27–36.
15. Snow K. Laci Peterson family endorses 'unborn victims' bill. Atlanta (GA): CNN Washington Bureau; 2003. Available at: http://www.cnn.com/2003/ALLPOLITICS/05/07/laci.bill/. Accessed June 12, 2015.
16. US Congress. Unborn Victims of Violence Act of 2004. Public Law 108–212 of 2004. Available at: https://www.congress.gov/bill/108th-congress/house-bill/1997/text. Accessed June 12, 2015.
17. Campbell JC. Abuse during pregnancy: a quintessential threat to maternal and child health - so when do we start to act? Can Med Assoc J 2001;164(11):1578–9.

Index

Note: Page numbers of article titles are in **boldface** type.

Crit Care Clin 32 (2016) 145–154
http://dx.doi.org/10.1016/S0749-0704(15)00098-6
0749-0704/16/$ – see front matter © 2016 Elsevier Inc. All rights reserved.

criticalcare.theclinics.com

Moving?

Make sure your subscription moves with you!

To notify us of your new address, find your **Clinics Account Number** (located on your mailing label above your name), and contact customer service at:

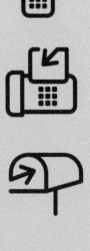

Email: journalscustomerservice-usa@elsevier.com

800-654-2452 (subscribers in the U.S. & Canada)
314-447-8871 (subscribers outside of the U.S. & Canada)

Fax number: 314-447-8029

Elsevier Health Sciences Division
Subscription Customer Service
3251 Riverport Lane
Maryland Heights, MO 63043

*To ensure uninterrupted delivery of your subscription, please notify us at least 4 weeks in advance of move.

Printed and bound by CPI Group (UK) Ltd, Croydon, CR0 4YY

03/10/2024

01040488-0014